LOVE
IN
LOVE
OUT

LOVE
IN
LOVE
OUT

A compassionate approach
to parenting your anxious child

DR MALIE COYNE

Thorsons

Thorsons
An imprint of HarperCollins*Publishers*
1 London Bridge Street
London SE1 9GF

www.harpercollins.co.uk

First published by Thorsons 2020

1 3 5 7 9 10 8 6 4 2

While the author of this work has made every effort to ensure that the information contained in this book is as accurate and up-to-date as possible at the time of publication, medical and pharmaceutical knowledge is constantly changing and the application of it to particular circumstances depends on many factors. Therefore it is recommended that readers always consult a qualified medical specialist for individual advice. This book should not be used as an alternative to seeking specialist medical advice which should be sought before any action is taken. The author and publishers cannot be held responsible for any errors and omissions that may be found in the text, or any actions that may be taken by a reader as a result of any reliance on the information contained in the text which is taken entirely at the reader's own risk.

In order to protect privacy, some names, identifying characteristics and details have been changed or reconstructed.

A catalogue record of this book is
available from the British Library

ISBN 978-0-00-833299-0

Printed and bound in Great Britain by
CPI Group (UK) Ltd, Croydon

MIX
Paper from
responsible sources
FSC™ C007454

To my beautiful girlies, Jessica and Aimée,
you make my heart smile.
And to my Pete xxx

The parent–child connection is the most powerful mental health intervention known to mankind.

Bessel van der Kolk

Contents

Author Biography

Dr Malie Coyne is a Clinical Psychologist and Psychology Lecturer at the National University of Ireland Galway and sits on the Mental Health Advisory Panel for the A Lust for Life charity. With her considerable experience of working with children and families, Malie is fast becoming one of the leading voices in compassionate parenting in Ireland. Through her advocacy work, public speaking and print, radio and television contributions, Malie shines a light on mental health issues and promotes well-being throughout our lives. Malie lives in Galway with her husband and two little ladies.

For more of her work, see www.drmaliecoyne.ie or follow Malie on social media.

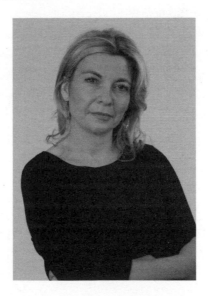

'We live in an age of anxiety. This book offers practical and evidence-based strategies to help parents navigate this new world. It is written by a parent for parents. *Love In, Love Out: A Compassionate Approach to Parenting Your Anxious Child* combines the best of psychological science with heartfelt and practical advice for parents who want to raise resilient children ready for the world.

This is one of those books to keep by the bedside; it's a go-to resource, a beacon of light and inspiration when the going gets tough as a parent in these anxious times we live in.'

– Dr Paul D'Alton,
Head of Psychology, St Vincent's University Hospital Dublin
Associate Professor of Psychology, University College Dublin
Fellow and former president, Psychological Society of Ireland

Foreword

Childhood is often referred to as the 'best years of your life', and children are often described as not having a care in the world – but that simply isn't true. Many children experience significant anxiety growing up. Sometimes it's rooted in their or their family's circumstances, but often a child's emotional maturity just isn't developed enough to process their little fears, be they rational or irrational. And anxiety can consume a child and limit their enjoyment of activities, their participation in school or social events and their quality of life.

Parents can struggle to understand or deal with their children's anxiety – sometimes allowing their own anxiety about their child's anxiety to make the situation worse.

Malie has created a road map for parents who are feeling lost or overwhelmed trying to help a child who is anxious. A clinical psychologist and parent who herself suffered with anxiety as a child, Malie has a warm, practical approach to dealing with the issue. She focuses on the use of calmness and compassion, which allow children to reason their way out of anxiety and to develop resilience. Her emphasis is on making an anxious child feel safe, secure and able to express their fear whilst empowering them to overcome it.

Using mindfulness and kindfulness, the benefits of play and cognitive-behaviour therapy this book will demonstrate to children and their parents that struggles in life are normal – and that they are necessary. Learning to master your anxiety and overcome its hold on you helps you to grow up stronger, more resilient and better capable of dealing with other struggles in life.

With simple, clear examples from her personal and professional experience throughout, *Love In, Love Out* is an invaluable aid to any family wanting their child to move beyond anxiety.

– Dr Ciara Kelly MB
Journalist, radio broadcaster and medical doctor

Introduction

What are your hopes for your children?

I'd like you to take a moment and ask yourself, 'What three qualities would I like my child to have?'

_____

_____

_____

If I only have one hope for my children, it's that they'll be compassionate. I've come to realise that being compassionate incorporates a lot of the qualities that many of us would wish for. This includes treating ourselves with kindness, having empathy towards others, engaging in meaningful and supportive relationships, showing gratitude, topped off by the icing on the cake commonly known as resilience.

Researchers are increasingly finding that the key to an emotionally healthy life is resilience. Resilience means learning to cope with manageable threats, while having the ability to rebound in the face of difficulties. Ultimately, it's about accepting life's colourful rainbow of emotions without becoming overwhelmed by them. The single most important factor that nurtures resilience in children is having a stable and committed relationship with a trusted adult, to whom the child can turn in times of challenge or need.

So, in building a child's resilience, the two primary ingredients are: facing a manageable threat and a secure child–parent relationship. Food for thought, isn't it?

As for the three qualities you picked for your children, I expect you came up with three words that match your values, background and current circumstances. There are no right or wrong answers to what you want for your children. But the fact remains that most parents have a rough idea of the qualities they would like to nurture in their kids.

An interesting follow-up question is:

Now think about what percentage of your time you spend intentionally developing these qualities in your children.

Don't worry – this question is not an attempt to make parents feel bad. Many parents spend much of their day just trying to survive, never mind putting effort into intentionally developing qualities in their children. For what it's worth, I don't wake up every morning thinking about the sorts of people I'd like my girlies to grow into, either!

What's important is learning to use precisely those occasions when you're trying to survive as a parent. These tough times will provide you with opportunities to help your children to thrive, giving you the chance to show them how to come out the other side when they're struggling with their worries. It's about trying to reframe these basic survival moments as times when the most important and most meaningful work of parenting actually takes place. This is called 'survive and thrive'.[1]

Any busy, stressed-out or disastrous episode in your week can become an opportunity for connection with your child. It's by connecting with you – rather than by having a perfect home life – that they can feel soothed, safe and cared for, and can begin to develop ways of soothing themselves. Similarly, every moment you invest in giving yourself time to reflect on your life and what influences you as a parent can become an opportunity for connection with your inner self and with those around you. Human connection heals adversity. It's as simple as that.

How to use this book

You've sought out this book to help you with your anxious child. But first, recognise what a worthy job you're already doing by being there for them, and how the relationship you've nurtured since the day they were born will be your greatest tool to see them through. I refer to 'parents' throughout the book, but the strategies presented are for any caregiver, or anyone who works with children. What's important to remember is that our role is crucial in preparing kids to live as human beings in this world, and managing life's inevitable highs and lows.

In looking at our role as parents, we'll kill off a couple of parenting myths. We'll firmly put to bed the idea of 'ideal' parenting – believe me, there ain't no such thing. Rather than see our kids as miniature versions of ourselves, we'll find a way of raising them without projecting our own problems and emotional baggage onto them. By doing this we'll learn to parent them without so much fear. I know it's a tall ask in this modern day, when fear is palpable all around us, but it's possible one step at a time.

When we understand our own and our children's anxiety, we realise that we're not alone in how we feel, that it's not our fault, and that it can get better with some help. It's not that we expect anxiety to go away completely, we just don't want it to stop us from doing the things we really enjoy doing to enable us to grow into emotionally healthy people.

The 'Anxiety made simple' sections throughout the book include answers to some of the questions I've been asked the most by children and parents. These provide simple explanations of some of the big questions about anxiety for you to share with your child as starting points for conversation.

Why you should talk to your child about anxiety

If you've opened this book because you're overwhelmed by your child's anxiety and want some practical ways of understanding and coping with it, that's exactly what this book is going to give you. But before we talk about the mechanics of anxiety, I need to make the following point loud and clear:

> Talking to your child about anxiety will not make them more anxious.

The reason I have a bee in my bonnet about this is that I've heard of several occasions in the past year when professional therapists have discouraged parents from broaching the subject of mental health with their teenage children. Some worry that by discussing stress and anxiety – or mental health more broadly – we'll make a bigger deal out of a small problem. Adults can have a tendency to shrug off children's concerns as being something they're picking up from their friends at school, and that by paying any attention to these concerns they might simply be giving them more traction.

• •

A case in point: Teresa

Teresa followed her previous therapist's advice and did not talk to her anxious teenage daughter, believing that she had caught this 'mental health' talk from her friends at school. Teresa was in a sense relieved, as she felt uncomfortable asking her daughter about her feelings. She was also afraid that asking about it might cause her daughter more anxiety and feared that her answer might be 'not good'. And what would she do then? But Teresa ultimately realised that in not asking the question, she was merely avoiding her own and her daughter's pain.

When we further explored Teresa's feelings and outlined the benefits of communicating versus not communicating her concerns, she felt more confident in broaching the issue with her daughter. She was also armed with the knowledge that teenagers are a special breed of people who do not like feeling under pressure to talk face to face. Bringing up concerns with teenagers is best done alone, side by side, in a car or when engaged in an activity, talking through the specifics of what the parent has noticed about the child's mood or behaviour:

> 'I've noticed you've been feeling sick before going to football the last few times, and that you have some scary thoughts about what might happen there. You also seem a bit frustrated about your school work, which is a new thing. Things seem tough for you at the moment. Is everything OK? Maybe talking would help, when you're ready. I'm here for you any time.'

By her next session with me, Teresa came in looking like a different woman. It was like a weight had been lifted off her shoulders. She said that it was only when she asked her daughter directly about her feelings that she had opened up:

'Unless I'd asked her directly how she was feeling, there's no way she would have opened up to me like she has this week. I knew there was something bothering her, but I didn't realise the extent of it. Now we can keep talking and figure out a way forward together.'

Teresa and her daughter still had a way to go from there, but she had made the first crucial step in letting her know that a) she had noticed her distress, that b) she was willing to sit with her daughter's pain and c) she wanted to help her through it.

• •

Some may think that it's best to leave it up to the child to bring up how they feel. The problem is that many kids – teenagers included – don't know how they feel or might not have the words to express it. They also don't have the benefit of your wisdom in detecting a change in their mood or behaviour, or connecting disparate events over time.

A child could also have caught on to the parent's reluctance to talk about feelings, and this might be preventing the child from being the first to speak up. Alternatively, a child might think a parent has enough on their plate as it is without them adding on their jumbled-up worries.

Consider this: what's the worst that can happen if you ask your child how they're feeling? You either hit the mark (they share what's going on) or you miss the mark (they tell you everything is fine – perhaps in their own unique way).

Whether it's a hit or a miss, by gently asking your child about what's going on inside them, you're opening up an important channel of communication. Sure, they may not use the opportunity today or even tomorrow, but keeping this channel open is vital for their emotional well-being. I call this 'speaking the language of feelings'. It can also involve you sharing your own experience of managing difficult feelings, so your child feels less alone with theirs.

I do appreciate that this and many of the ideas in this book will come more easily to some parents than others, but working through the steps in this book should help both you and your child. This book is intended as a source of ideas and encouragement, one that can be dipped into in anxious times, but each section can also be read in turn. By first introducing compassion followed by anxiety I intend to give us a shared understanding of what we're dealing with. Then, by focusing on parents, I'm acknowledging the importance of parents stepping back, taking a breath and reflecting on themselves and their own stresses. From there, we can then take a look at what your anxious child might be feeling, and move on to real, practical exercises for everyday life with a compassionate and hopeful approach to managing anxiety for both you and your child.

1
What is Compassion?

Love in, love out

My friend Ruth is just like you and me. She loves her kids to bits. Tries her best. Feels overwhelmed by their needs sometimes, reacts in frustration, wishes she hadn't, feels guilty, tries to learn from it, gets back up again and tries her best all over again. Rinse and repeat.

What I love about Ruth is how she makes me feel OK to be a full of love, imperfect mama. Because that's what she is and I love her for it. I first met her when we were lying in beds across from each other in the postnatal ward right after having our second babies. There we were, complete strangers struggling with pure exhaustion, rollercoaster emotions, and feeling very vulnerable. Isn't it amazing how vulnerability opens us up to human connection like that?

Ruth and I often talk about our many parenting challenges and mess-ups. One day she shared this beautiful affirmation with me, which she uses to ground herself during really tough moments with her children. It goes:

Love in (take a deep breath in) …
(pause, hold your breath) …
Love out (deep breath out)

When I first heard her affirmation I was instantly drawn to it. I thought, 'Well, if Ruth finds it helpful, then maybe I could use it too when I'm having a shit-hard parenting moment.' Times like these are so overwhelming, surely anything is worth a try!

Inhaling *Love in* and exhaling *Love out* makes us press pause. We take a moment to recognise how hard it is to be a parent, before we press play again to respond to our children's feelings. Being kind to ourselves makes us better able to be kind to those we love the most.

The importance of compassion comes through loud and clear – we need to give ourselves a break, so that we can give our kids a break. Take a moment for ourselves so that we can give our child the warmth and understanding that he or she needs. If we take that step back – remembering that we *all* experience stressful times with children – we can refocus our attention on being supportive and caring towards them.

Better still, when you accompany the deep breath in and out with a physical gesture of warmth and care, like putting your hands over your heart or over your belly, your bonding hormone (oxytocin) is released with your touch and the toxic stress hormone (cortisol) is reduced.

It struck me that *Love in, love out* could be an affirmation that any parent could use, especially those struggling to manage their children's big feelings – and their own.

Of course, that's not to say that we'll always have it in us to take a breath, let alone pause and reflect during those really overwhelming moments, but it may just remind us that if a moment is really hard, it will pass – and that we all deserve compassion, most of all from ourselves.

Our own worst critics

We all have it in ourselves to be very self-critical, especially when things aren't going well: '*Why* is this happening to us?'; 'My kid *shouldn't* do this'; 'I *ought* to be able to handle this.' Thinking like this – which we all do at times – doesn't accept the reality of the situation and places unhelpful expectations on everyone. Difficult times do happen. It's how we deal with them that counts.

So, when we hear that critical voice, we calmly acknowledge its presence and allow a kinder voice to gently break through the surface. Just as we would comfort a close friend going through a tough moment, if we can learn to treat ourselves kindly through our parenting struggles, then everything else becomes a lot easier.

Like a hug from a friend, being kinder to ourselves helps us to combat stress and to release our brain's feel-good chemical, serotonin. This helps to lift our mood and activate our coping skills, increasing the likelihood that we'll reach out to others for support.

This 'self-compassion' has been dubbed the 'newest parenting skill', though in truth there's nothing very new about it, as it's based on age-old scientific evidence as to how we, as mammals, react to comfort:

> One of the things unique to mammals is that we are programmed to respond to warmth, gentle touch and soft vocalisations. That's what keeps vulnerable infants close to their mothers and safe from harm. So when we provide that kind of touch and calm reassurance to ourselves, we actually reduce levels of stress hormones and boost the feel-good ones. Then we feel safe, comforted and in the optimal frame of mind to do our best.[2]

So there you go. *Love in, love out* – spoken softly with warmth, accompanied by gentle in-and-out breathing and soothing touch – could be our gift of kindness to ourselves. Breathing in and out of the place of frustration, grounding ourselves before choosing our response, is both kind to ourselves and, ultimately, kind to others.[3]

Self-compassion is helpful for parents when we find ourselves struggling with our children's emotions because:

- It helps us to face up to what's happening in the tougher moments and acknowledge that we're having trouble coping: 'This is a moment of struggle with my child. This is really hard right now. But it's OK.'
- It helps us to be kind in how we think about the situation and acknowledge our common experience in facing difficulties: 'Struggles with our kids are a part of life. Many children have worries. Other parents find it hard to manage, and they feel the same way as I do.'
- We need to treat ourselves with kindness as we would a good friend in the same situation – with gentleness, warmth, patience and encouragement: 'May I be kind to myself in this moment.'
- With this kindness, we can take action, because compassion is best understood as something that we do in response to a difficult situation: '*Love in* for myself; *love out* towards my child, and bringing calm and connection to this difficult moment.'[4,5]

Taking a minute to reset

An alternative meaning to *Love in, love out* came from one of my writing mentors. He interpreted it as a mantra involving the power of the breath to calm us down by switching our brain's fight-flight-freeze mode to a gentler, more rational mode. He liked that peaceful, rhythmic quality about it: *Love in, love out. Love in, love out.* It's a soothing message of compassion for you – and your child.

Originally derived from Hinduism and Buddhism, a mantra is a word, phrase or sound believed to have a special spiritual power, which is repeated to aid concentration in meditation or prayer and expresses a strong belief. A mantra is a great tool for both parents and children to encourage us to press pause on a difficult situation or to spur us on when we need a good boost.

Because our inner voice has huge power over how we feel about ourselves and how we make sense of and respond to our experiences, compassionate mantras like *Love in, love out* balance the negative inner voice we often tune into during our hardest moments.

Many of us – and especially parents – are grandmasters at beating ourselves up at every opportunity we get. Being nice to ourselves may feel really alien to some of us. It's as if we think that being hard on ourselves will keep us 'in line' and make us better parents. On the contrary; being self-critical doesn't prevent bad things from happening, and it can actually make things worse for both us and our kids.

Being self-critical can be really harmful to both our emotional and physical health and is linked to everything from depression to anxiety to high blood pressure to a general sense of dissatisfaction with life. Just like a physical attack sends our brain's fight-flight-freeze response into overdrive, so does an emotional attack, even if we're directing it at ourselves.[6] At times, modern-day man's worst predator can be himself.

To add insult to injury, when we engage in self-criticism, not only are we the 'attacked' but we're also the 'attacker' – making the process doubly exhausting. With all this going on in our brains, no wonder self-criticism can lead to anxiety. To make matters worse, self-criticism can also *arise* from anxiety. This is because people with anxiety can feel alone in their pain and powerless to do anything about it, and they criticise themselves for it.

Mantras are in essence the antidote to our brain's age-old tendency towards negativity and they ensure that self-kindness trumps self-blame. I'm down with that. It's about being mindful of how you talk to – and about – yourself, because your words are powerful.[7] Examples include: 'Breathe'; 'It's OK'; 'This shall pass'; 'It is what it is'; 'Try a hug'; 'Namaste'; or whichever other positive words float your boat!

Practising being positive about ourselves, to ourselves, is a hell of a lot easier when all is rosy in the family garden, when your kids are getting along and are in a good emotional place. But it's actually during the most challenging moments, when our kids are highly emotional and are testing our patience, that taking a mindful pause is one of the best tools you can hone. We may not be able to control their out-of-control behaviour, but we can try our best to respond to them in a calmer way.

Compassion 'in' and 'out' trays

Love in, love out can also be seen as a poignant offering from parents to their children.[8]

Think of the 'in' and 'out' trays you'd find in an office. If a parent focuses on putting *love in* to their child, the child is then enabled to give *love out* to themselves, their parents, families, friends, teachers and communities. That's a lot of 'outs' for one 'in', isn't it?

This is why the child–parent relationship is so important in making a child feel safe, comfortable in their own skin, able to manage big feelings and show compassion towards others. When we put *love in* to a child it builds a strong foundation for the child to develop compassion for themselves, to nurture important social and emotional connections, and to grow life-long resilience.

With all these meanings attached to it, *Love in, love out* grew into something pretty special for me. That is what I intend to offer you in this book. If I can pour my heart into you and your parenting through sharing my vulnerabilities and the wisdom my clients have gifted me with, then *Love in, love out* may hopefully become something special for you too.

 If you'd like to try a *Love in, love out* meditation, flip ahead to page 252.

Why a compassionate approach?

I was a little stressed myself while I was preparing to contribute to a TV documentary exploring our modern-day experience of stress[9] – the irony! I was trying to decide which therapeutic approach would be most helpful for father-of-one Jonathan, and was more than a little nervous about my skills in psychology being exposed on camera in front of the whole nation.

I wanted to choose the best approach to help Jonathan to feel less stressed and overwhelmed in his daily life. The goal was for him to focus on what mattered most to him, such as his connection with his family and living more in the moment.

But I needn't have worried about my performance. Compassion did its thing, and I felt like the privileged messenger.

It being television, the production team would have preferred me to come up with a therapeutic process that was more visual: daring him to jump off a diving board, for instance, or taking a relaxing walk through a beautiful meadow. Instead, Jonathan's journey of self-discovery took its natural course when we began to focus on compassion.

The healing properties of compassion have been celebrated for centuries. Compassion has always been considered a vital quality by both Western and Eastern philosophies and religions, and now even has its own therapy called 'compassion-focused therapy', which is gaining a following among psychologists, psychiatrists and other medical professionals.

 To find out more about compassionate parenting in action, flip ahead to page 125.

The origin of the word 'compassion' reveals its powerful meaning and significance. *Compati* in Latin is 'suffer with', so 'compassion' is, by definition, relational; that is, it requires a relationship with the people around us. Compassion requires sharing in the experience of suffering – and if we accept that there is suffering to be had, we're recognising that the human experience – life – is imperfect.

Compassion is the realisation that all human beings make mistakes, have regrets, and struggle with feelings of inadequacy and disappointment – and that we're all in the same boat together. Knowing this somehow brings comfort:

> The pain I feel in difficult times is the same pain you feel in difficult times. The triggers are different, the circumstances are different, the degree of pain is different, but the process is the same. You can't always get what you want. This is true for everyone, even the Rolling Stones.[10]

To have compassion for others, you must first notice that they're suffering, then be moved by their suffering, and feel warmth and caring and a desire to help them. When they make mistakes, you offer understanding and kindness, rather than judgement.

Compassion not only involves a sensitivity to our own and other people's distress, but a motivation to prevent or alleviate it.[11] Being compassionate means that someone else's pain becomes your pain, and that crucially, you take steps to do something about it.

Having compassion for yourself during hard moments – like when you're raising your children – means watching out for how you're feeling, and treating yourself with the same kindness and understanding you'd give others. It also means seeing failures as part of the human condition, and having a balanced awareness of painful thoughts and emotions.

Self-compassion is just as important in improving our overall health as having compassion for others, with multiple studies showing that greater self-compassion is linked to less anxiety and depression.[12] One of the reasons for this is that self-compassionate people are more likely to accept their emotions without judgement and are less likely to worry than those who lack self-compassion.[13]

Accepting our imperfections with kindness appears to break the cycle of negativity and deactivates the body's fight-flight-freeze response.

Compassion is a foundation for sharing our aliveness and building a more humane world.[14]

Like the ripple created by throwing a pebble in a pond, one act of compassion can have an effect that may reach around the world.[15] If one single act of compassion can have such an impact, imagine the potential impact of parents being compassionate towards themselves on a regular basis. As they witness their parents emerging calmer and more confident, the ripple will affect these children's own relationships with themselves and others.

Many parents I meet are stuck in patterns of self-blame and feel powerless to help their children who are struggling with their big feelings, be they anxiety, grief, anger, sadness, guilt or shame. The truth is that parents are often struggling with big feelings of their own. Big feelings meeting big feelings is not an easy combination!

If we could somehow bring compassion into common parenting struggles we might shift how parents and children view their problems and how well they think they can cope. Because it's not about our actual ability to cope, is it? It's usually more about how we think we'll cope in any given situation, which then affects our feelings and our responses. Not only does anxiety narrow our focus and make us overestimate the size of the problem at hand, it leads us to underestimate our ability to cope with that problem.

Naturally, parents who come into my clinic are looking for my perspective on what is happening with their child and suggestions on how to best help them. I find that teasing out how the parents feel in response to their child's big feelings is usually the best first step.

Listening and being compassionate, parent to parent, is the best gift I can offer them. Naturally, I'll have my opinion on their difficulties and have tools in my toolbox to share with parents, but the most important thing is to build a relationship so they feel more comfortable with the journey we're embarking on together.

And that is why I'm using the compassionate approach as a foundation for supporting you in helping your anxious child. It provides the scaffolding needed to support you and your child to feel safe, connected and empowered.

Compassion-focused therapy
and the Three Circles

> Compassion reduces our fear, boosts our confidence, and
> opens us to inner strength. By reducing distrust, it opens
> us to others and brings us a sense of connections with
> them and a sense of purpose and meaning in life.
>
> *Dalai Lama*

Compassion-focused therapy (CFT)[16] pays particular attention
to how our early childhood experiences have affected the types
of emotions we have as adults. It's especially useful for people
who are particularly critical of themselves or who have high
levels of shame, as well as people who have difficulty feeling
warmth towards, and being kind to, themselves or others. For
adults and children alike, these problems are often rooted in
a difficult childhood in which the child may not have felt safe,
loved or valued as much as they needed.

CFT deals with the ways that we learn to manage our
emotions from childhood onwards. Research in neuroscience
shows that humans have evolved at least three types of
emotional regulation system – or Three Circles, as they're
known – that work together to control and maintain our
emotions. These Three Circles help us to navigate and understand our emotional world and that of our children. Looking
at these is helpful for both parents and children because they
help to explain the guiding forces behind our reactions to the
daily challenges we face.

If you look at the diagram on page 20,[17] the three systems are:

- The Threat system – helps us to detect and respond to
  threats in our lives. If the Threat system had a motto, it
  would be 'better safe than sorry'. It's commonly associated

with anger, fear, anxiety, guilt, disgust and our inner self-critic.

- The Drive system – enables us to go out and get what we need, and to take pleasure in doing it. It's what helps to get you out of bed in the mornings, and is connected with desire, the thrill of the chase, achievement and excitement.
- The Soothing system – helps to calm and nurture us and to balance the other two systems. It gives us positive feelings of peaceful well-being, safety, connection and contentment.

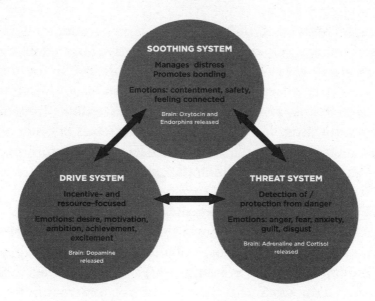

The diagram of the Three Circles shows how one system can dominate over another, with Threat often taking over while Soothing goes undernourished. Both the Threat and Soothing circles can feed into the Drive circle. The diagram helps you to understand which aspects of your life typically fit into each of the circles:

Threat: any major pressure in any area of your life – be it at work, in your relationships, among your family. Anything that threatens your sense of worth and safety.

Drive: anything that motivates you to get up in the morning, whether positive or negative.

Soothing: what you enjoy doing; passions; positive relationships; hobbies; what you do in your downtime. Whatever makes you feel safe.

By paying particular attention to whichever system is less active, we can learn to manage each system more effectively. Nurturing the underactive circle reduces symptoms such as low mood, anxiety and stress, and helps us to respond to everyday situations in an emotionally healthier way.

CFT focuses on the link between our thoughts, how we live our lives and our Three Circles. Through activities like attention training and mindfulness, compassionate skills are cultivated to help clients notice how their minds can be taken over by negative emotions and to nurture their relationship with themselves and with others.

CFT is a wonderful therapy for managing many mental health and emotional issues. This is particularly true for stress and anxiety, which occur when the body's Threat and Drive systems are going hell for leather at the expense of an underactive Soothing system. Indeed the modern-world experience of toxic stress may have its origins in not feeling good enough in childhood, which manifests in later life as a greatly reduced Soothing circle, triggering a Threat reaction related to the fear of rejection or abandonment.[18]

CFT helps people to develop the resources to deal with difficult emotions. The beauty of it is that it enables them to disclose deeper feelings, such as unworthiness and shame, which other psychological therapies can have a hard time targeting. Handling such feelings productively prevents us from compensating with behaviours such as working, eating or exercising to excess, or resorting to drugs or alcohol.

The three qualities of self-compassion

We have already caught glimpses of how useful self-compassion can be in approaching anxiety in children and adults. Derived from pioneering psychological research,[19] the three central qualities of self-compassion are self-kindness, our shared human experience and mindfulness, which combine and interact to improve our state of mind. Below is a list that compares these three qualities to their opposites, showing how much more useful self-compassion is for helping us and our children with the challenges we all face:

- **Self-kindness versus self-judgement:** Working on being kind to yourself and less judgemental is easier said than done, isn't it? In building our emotional reserves as parents, we need to be more accepting of our own limits, and learn to step away from negative feelings about ourselves. In being a little kinder to ourselves, we'll be calmer, more balanced and better able to care for ourselves and our children.

- **Common humanity versus isolation:** If we feel that we're the only person struggling with a particular problem, we'll end up feeling isolated. But if we recognise that suffering, relationship troubles and mistakes are part of being human, we're far more likely to open ourselves up to connecting with other people, to forgive ourselves and others, and to get back up and try again!

- **Mindfulness versus over-identification:** Those who suffer with anxiety often focus on the past and the future, and feel both weighing heavily upon them. Mindfulness is a powerful tool for both children and their parents in navigating the storms of anxiety. When we accept our emotions rather than judge ourselves for being emotional, our emotions tend to run their natural and relatively short-lived course.[20]

The healing balm of self-compassion

When we soothe our painful feelings with the healing balm of self-compassion, not only are we changing our mental and emotional experience, we're also changing our body chemistry.[21]

By tapping into our body's self-healing Soothing system we trigger the release of oxytocin. Known as 'the hormone of love', and particularly associated with first cuddles between parents and newborns, this chemical helps us to feel safe, calm and securely connected with others. Oxytocin is responsible for fine-tuning our brain's social instincts and making us do things to strengthen close relationships.

Oxytocin is released in a variety of social situations, from when a baby is first held, to when parents joyfully interact with their children, to when someone you really love gives you a hug – when released it makes you more likely to feel warmth and compassion for yourself and empathy towards others.

> Because thoughts and emotions have the same impact
> on our bodies irrespective of whether they're directed
> towards ourselves or others, self-compassion is a
> powerful trigger for the release of oxytocin.[22]

But wait for it: our dear friend oxytocin is actually a stress hormone that your pituitary gland pumps out as part of your biological stress response. Just as the stress hormone cortisol is released to spur you into immediate action and adrenaline is released to make your heart pound, oxytocin is released in response to a perceived threat so you notice when someone close is struggling or to motivate you to seek support and be surrounded by those who care about you. Amazing isn't it?

In her groundbreaking book *The Upside of Stress* and her TED talk 'How to make stress your friend',[23] health psychologist Kelly McGonigal talks about the impact of our beliefs about stress on our overall health. According to McGonigal, our bodies have a built-in mechanism to help us cope with stress: the human connection.

Stress gives us access to our hearts. The compassionate heart that finds joy and meaning in connecting with others, and yes, your pounding physical heart, working so hard to give you strength and energy, and when you choose to view stress in this way, you're not just getting better at stress, you're actually making a pretty profound statement. You're saying that you can trust yourself to handle life's challenges, and you're remembering that you don't have to face them alone.

McGonigal supports the idea that the quality and power of our Soothing systems are strongly associated with the bonds we form with others from early childhood onwards, a concept that's also central to attachment theory.[24] In human beings, the first and most powerful bond an infant is programmed to make is usually with their mother or father. This attachment serves to improve the baby's chance of survival (think food, comfort and our most basic needs) when faced with a threat, brings a sense of mutual connection and well-being, and builds the foundation for virtually every aspect of the child's development.

> Talking about attachment and childhood can trigger painful memories and thoughts for many parents, myself included. Please be mindful of this as you read this book and gain support from close loved ones – or a professional – if you're struggling. You may not have expected to go so deep, but as my own counsellor told me after a tough session, 'Once you hit the bottom of the pool, you can only bounce back up.'

Galway City Early Years Committee and the Galway Parent Network ran a poster campaign that was based on this idea called 'How to build a happy baby' as part of an infant mental health initiative. We don't often think of the mental health of babies, but it refers to a child's social and emotional development from birth to age three within the context of their relationship with the most important person in their lives.

Based on the UNICEF and the World Health Organization (WHO) Baby Friendly Health Initiative,[25] we created four posters containing simple, positively framed, evidence-based messages emphasising the innate abilities of human beings to look after their babies. The purpose of the posters was to promote the importance of the child–parent attachment and to dispel common parenting myths.[26] One read:

> New babies have a strong need to be close to their parents, as this helps them to feel secure and loved, like they matter in the world.
>   **Myth:** Babies become spoilt and demanding if they're given too much attention.
>   **Truth:** When babies' needs for love and comfort are met, they'll be calmer and grow up to be more confident.
>   **Evidence:** Close skin-to-skin body contact, postnatally and beyond, significantly improves the physical and mental health and well-being for both mother and baby. When babies feel secure, they release a hormone called oxytocin, which acts like a fertiliser for their growing brain, helping them to be happier and more confident as they grow older. Holding, smiling and talking to your baby also releases oxytocin in you, which also has a soothing effect.[27]

Crucially, the child–parent attachment bond that we all see in babies remains strong for child and parent as they grow older. The first three years of life, when a child's brain develops the fastest, are a critical window of opportunity for establishing a healthy stress response, although it's never too late to help your child to manage their distress.

Soothing your child during their stressful or anxious moments releases oxytocin in both of you, giving child and parent a sense of security and helping you to become more resilient, knowing that your bond with each other is strong. When you tune in to your child's feelings and help them to calm down, you also play a significant role in easing their fears and their fight-flight-freeze cortisol levels.

A parent's compassionate response to their child during their anxious moments has the power to deactivate their Threat system and activate their Soothing system. The calmer and safer a child feels, the more open and flexible they'll be in response to their environments and the more likely they'll be able to use the tools to evaluate and manage future threats.

Relationships like the one you share with your child work to transform 'stress and anxiety into catalysts for courage and connection'.[28] While anxiety is certainly not a pleasant experience for anyone, it might help to know that your child has a naturally strong desire to connect with you during their most anxious moments, even though it may not always appear that way.

2
What is Anxiety?

In this age of ever-growing anxiety, it's becoming increasingly difficult for the average parent to know what is a healthy level of anxiety in their children, and what is something to be more concerned about. Our kids face a multitude of challenges at all stages of their development: from toddlers with nightmares, to primary school children with separation anxiety and tummy pains, to self-conscious adolescents who find social situations terrifying.

Anxieties are common in childhood, and are often part and parcel of growing up. Everyone experiences anxiety, which is a product of our 'tricky' survival brains[29] trying to cope with life's constantly changing demands. A useful way of looking at anxiety is as a simple formula: add up all the things that cause our children stress, and then subtract their beliefs about their ability to cope. The net result is their anxiety level.[30] So it's how a child *copes* with their anxiety that marks the difference between them thriving in their daily lives or having real difficulty meeting new experiences with open arms.

Your response to your child's anxiety is a crucial factor in how your child will cope. With their supportive guidance, parents like you hold the key to anchoring their children with safety and connection. From this strong foundation, you and your child can work on problem-solving strategies together to help alleviate their anxiety.

That is why it's so important for you to be able to recognise when anxiety is beginning to affect your child's daily life and their ability to function.

Anxiety made simple

Question: What is anxiety, and is it normal?

Answer: Everyone feels anxious sometimes. It's normal to feel a bit anxious when you're meeting someone new, when you've just got on a rollercoaster, when you've been asked to speak in class or are waiting just before a test. Just like adults, some kids feel it only a bit, while others feel it a lot more.

When anxiety comes, you'll know that something doesn't feel quite right, but you may not have the words to explain what's happening to you. This is particularly true for children and teenagers. You may feel like something bad might happen to you or to someone you care about. You might also be angry or sad and want to avoid doing things, or simply wish to stay at home.

Anxiety is the body's alarm system that has always helped human beings to survive. It works so well that it kicks in even when it's not needed, like when we believe there is danger when there is none, or when we start to ask ourselves 'What if' something terrible happens.

People who are feeling anxious are scanning for danger, and are mega alert to the body's alarm signals. That's why anxiety can feel so exhausting!

Anxiety is not a sign of anything being wrong or of being weak. It's a sign that your strong, healthy brain is doing exactly what it's meant to do to protect you from danger. Anxiety doesn't care if the threat is real or imagined, because our brain would rather keep us safe than be sorry.

Sometimes our brain goes overboard in trying to protect us. When this happens, it sets off a chain reaction of nasty feelings in our bodies. Feeling bad makes us think anxious thoughts, which makes us even more anxious, like a vicious circle. It's as if we're ready for action, but there's no enemy, so tension builds up in our bodies without having a chance to be let out!

Anxiety as a problem

Anxiety becomes a problem when it affects a child's sense of who they are, their relationships and their engagement with school and other activities. Anxiety becomes a problem when a child's worries – whether their thoughts, feelings or physical sensations – are making them avoid situations, which in turn restricts their learning and enjoyment of life.

Distinguishing anxiety from normal fears is important. Throughout childhood, we all naturally experience transient fears that arise in line with our ability to recognise and understand potential dangers in our environment.

When a child is young, fears seem to be immediate and tangible, like separation from a loved one or a fear of strangers. As the child gets older, fears seem to become more abstract, centring on thoughts that anticipate problems ('what if?') and focusing on the less tangible (bad dreams, someone getting hurt, or struggling at school).[31] Children are expected to 'grow out of' many of these fears as they develop.

Sadly, this is more difficult for some children than for others, which is why it's important to focus on what is happening in your child's world. If you feel that anxiety is having a significant impact on your child's daily life and ability to function, then it may be time to seek some professional support in guiding you and your child forward.

Basic symptoms of anxiety

Many children have the problems listed below at some point, but if your child has been struggling with one or more of these symptoms more days than not for the past six months, it may be time to talk to your GP.

Your GP can advise you about reputable local support services. These might include a psychologist, psychotherapist, play therapist or counsellor.

- Excessive anxiety and worry about a number of events or activities
- Worry that is hard to control
- Restlessness or feeling keyed up or on edge
- Becoming easily fatigued
- Difficulty concentrating or mind going blank
- Irritability
- Muscle tension
- Sleep problems: difficulty falling or staying asleep, restlessness, or unsatisfying sleep
- Difficulties in school, in social settings, dealing with others[32]

Your doctor will also want to rule out other potential causes of anxiety, including medical conditions, the side-effects of medication, drug or alcohol use, and any other mental health concerns.

Adrenaline and our bodies[33]

There are very real reasons why your body feels the way it does when you're anxious. When there's nothing to fight or run away from, there's nothing to burn up the fight-flight-freeze fuel – adrenaline – that's rushing through your body.

Adrenaline is a stress hormone whose job it is to get you up and moving, often for positive reasons, like excitement, meeting a deadline or running a race. This big boost of energy helps us to do our best. But adrenaline also rushes into our bodies when we're feeling anxious, worried or threatened, when there's no deadline to meet or race to run, so there's nowhere for it to go.

Here are some of the things you might feel when adrenaline builds up and why you might feel them when you're anxious:

1. Shallow and fast breath

What's happening? Your brain tells your body to stop wasting oxygen – instead of using it on strong, deep breaths, your body is told to send it to the muscles so they can fight or run away.

How you might feel. Your breathing changes from strong, slow, deep breaths to fast, little breaths. You might feel puffed or a bit breathless. Your cheeks might blush red and your face might feel warm.

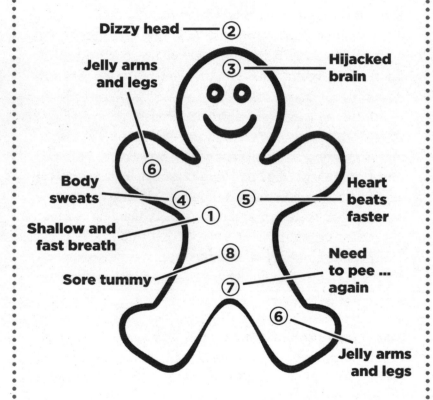

Dizzy head ── ②

Jelly arms
and legs

③ Hijacked
brain

Body
sweats ④

⑥

⑤ Heart
beats
faster

①

Shallow and
fast breath

Sore tummy

⑧

Need
to pee ...
again

⑦

⑥

Jelly arms
and legs

2. Dizzy head
What's happening? If you don't fight or run away, levels of oxygen build up in your body and carbon dioxide levels drop from all that fast breathing.

How you might feel. Dizzy, confused or sick.

3. Hijacked brain
What's happening? When you have an anxious adrenaline rush, other feelings such as anger or sadness might turn up to high volume as well. When your thoughts are racing, it's hard to think clearly with the logical, calming part of your brain, the prefrontal cortex.

How you might feel. Angry or sad, as though you want to burst into tears, sometimes for no reason at all. Your 'wise leader' – the prefrontal cortex – shuts down.

4. Body sweats
What's happening? Your body cools itself down by sweating so it doesn't overheat if you have to fight or run away.

How you might feel. Clammy or sweaty, even if it's cold out.

5. Heart beats faster
What's happening? Your heart beats faster and your pulse rises to get the oxygen around your body, especially to the arms and legs, allowing you to run away or attack.

How you might feel. Your heart can feel like it's racing and you might also feel sick. This can feel scary, like a heart attack. It's OK, though – you're perfectly safe.

6. Jelly arms and legs

What's happening? Fuel gets sent to your bigger muscles in the arms (in case you need to fight) and the legs (in case you need to run away).

How you might feel. Your arms and legs might feel tight or wobbly.

7. Need to pee ... again

What's happening? Adrenaline can make you want to pee. We know it happens, but we don't really know why.

How you might feel. As if your bladder's full and you want to empty it.

8. Sore tummy

What's happening? The digestive system shuts down so the fuel it was using to digest food can be used by your arms and legs in case you have to fight or run away.

How you might feel. As if there are butterflies in your tummy. You might also feel sick, as if you're going to vomit – and your mouth might feel a bit dry.

With all these things happening in your body, no wonder you might feel exhausted, shaky and weak after the adrenaline has died down!

The causes of anxiety

Finding the causes of a child's problematic anxiety can be complicated. They can often assume the form of an interweaving web that might take quite some time to untangle. Sometimes the root causes of anxiety aren't as clear as we'd like them to be, but that doesn't mean that an anxious child won't benefit hugely from our compassion, anchoring support and the approaches outlined in this book.

Common reasons for difficulty coping with anxiety range from a child's unique temperament or personality, to what a child has gleaned from observing their parents and key adults, the presence of any traumatic events or 'anxiety triggers' in their lives, all the way to being vulnerable to the impact of the wider society in which they live.

All these interacting factors at play can make it extremely difficult for children to share their anxious feelings, for parents to navigate the best way forward, for teachers to respond appropriately, and for doctors, therapists and others to support children and their families.

Many of the parents I meet are hugely eager to *find a reason* for their child's anxiety so that they can begin to make helpful changes to their environment and identify the most appropriate ways to support them.

Of course it can certainly help to know what triggers your child's anxiety and what eases it, so you can better equip them with the tools to identify and manage it. But a vital precursor to introducing these problem-solving tools into your child's life is the role you as a parent play in anchoring them back to safety during their wobbly moments, which crucially involves you feeling calm and nurtured in the first instance.

However, I would urge you not to fixate on trying to find a reason for your child's anxiety, as it may not always be clear.

What's more important is to take each day as it comes, and to respond calmly to your child's emotions with empathy and compassion in the moment.

> Regardless of the specific reason or reasons for your child's anxiety, the experience of anxiety itself is quite similar in everyone. This is simply because as human beings we all share the same survival response to threatening situations, which negatively impacts our thoughts, feelings, body sensations and behaviour. Whilst the intensity of this response can vary between humans, the feeling of anxiety is universal.
>
> For that reason the techniques I introduce in this book apply to *any* child *of any age*, irrespective of the reasons why they may be anxious.

Although the experience of anxiety is much the same for everyone, we're now experiencing unprecedented levels of anxiety throughout our lives. Why is that, and how can we reduce the impact of negative social factors on children's well-being?

The Age of Anxiety

We had the Stone Age, the Iron Age, the Bronze Age, the Industrial Age and the Technological Age. Now we have the Age of Anxiety. Why do I say that? We are bombarded with messages from the world about all the things that are dangerous, could be dangerous or will be dangerous.[34]

Anxiety is rife among children today, and I've seen a massive increase in the number of children being referred to me with this condition in recent years. Even though anxiety is the most common mental health issue facing children in the Western world today[35] and the most prevalent psychological disorder in schoolchildren, it has been described as a 'silent epidemic' as it can often go undetected and untreated.

Because children who suffer from anxiety don't necessarily draw attention to themselves and often present as well behaved, they can frequently be left to suffer in silence as they're overlooked or mistaken for being shy. Some children might act out angrily in an effort to cope with their hidden anxious feelings, which may also lead to misunderstanding, while others hide their anxiety behind a veil of perfectionism, petrified of doing anything wrong or of making the tiniest mistake.

Anxiety hides behind many masks, which cover up a multitude of scary thoughts. A child hiding their anxiety can be really lonely, as they continue to suffer while concealing their real self from the world. A child's real self can be itching to get out – if only they knew how or had the courage to let it happen. Being isolated like this also means that the child is alone with their own thoughts, usually preoccupied with something that happened in the past or that might happen in the future, which makes it hard for them to live in the moment.

Although we have a better standard of living than previous generations, and have come on leaps and bounds in terms of our health care, we still have a very long way to go. The irony is that the world we now live in is actually *contributing* to anxiety for both parents and children. The demands of the world are increasing, which makes us feel threatened and shakes our faith in our ability to cope.

Deciding what's important:
different kinds of goals

One of the ways in which the world we live in makes us anxious can be related to the kinds of goals we choose to pursue. Some goals are bigger-picture; others are very specific.

An *intrinsic goal* is one very much related to the activity that achieves it, where the enjoyment comes from the journey as opposed to the end result. Intrinsic goals include spending quality time with loved ones, living life according to one's values, pursuing a dream, or anything that gives life meaning.

On the other hand, an *extrinsic goal* is distantly related to the activities that achieve them which are often seen as imposed by the outside world. Examples include achieving high marks in school, winning sports games, achieving high status and looking a certain way.

There has been a continual shift away from intrinsic goals in our pressurised modern world in favour of extrinsic goals. This is to our detriment, as the pursuit of extrinsic at the expense of intrinsic goals has been linked to increased rates of anxiety and depression. This makes sense, as what we do to pursue extrinsic goals is often less satisfying than when we follow our intrinsic goals. What's more, we often have less control over how successfully we meet our extrinsic goals for the simple reason that they rely on external forces. An over-emphasis on extrinsic goals is linked to an overactive Threat system feeding our Drive system; on the other hand, enjoying the process of meeting our intrinsic goals nurtures our Soothing system, leading to more positive Drive in our lives.

Our Drive system is frequently over-stimulated because we live in a society that encourages us to want more, to have more and to be more.[36] This 'scarcity culture' occurs when everyone is hyper-aware of what they lack:

Everything from safety and love to money and resources feels restricted or lacking. We spend inordinate amounts of time calculating how much we have, want and don't have and how much everyone else has, needs and wants.[37]

Our caveman brains and the negativity bias

Our Age of Anxiety is, in great part, the result of trying to do today's jobs with yesterday's tools![38]

Our brains haven't changed much if at all since the human race began, but the kinds of threats we face have. Back in the days of the caveman, when human beings were presented with many more physical dangers, it was our brains that helped us to survive basic and very tangible threats, such as predators.

Our brains have always tricked us by overestimating threats and comparing us unfavourably to others – they do this to keep us safe. If we think things are worse than they are – and that we're at greater risk than we are – we'll be more careful and have a better chance of survival.

Part of the reason that we're still afraid of what might happen to us, and hyper-aware of what we lack, is because of this age-old trick that our brains play on us in order to protect us. This also includes our inner critical voice, ever present to give its opinion at the drop of a hat.

Incredibly, for every negative thing that happens, we need five positives to balance it out! This is where making a conscious effort to be kind to ourselves and others comes into play.

But why does this kind of negative focus have so much staying power? The *negativity bias* – our natural tendency to attend to and respond more readily to negative information – is a very real force determining how we behave, and has been found in babies as young as three months old. Our collective negativity bias arises from both innate predispositions and our learned experience: nature and nurture combined.

Our negativity bias plays a significant role in our views about ourselves, our emotions, our ability to take in information and our decision-making. Left unchecked, it can become a serious impediment to good mental health, as it has been found to be synonymous with anxiety and depression.[39]

Modern technology meets tricky brain

Our contemporary epidemic of anxiety arises from trying to cope with today's challenges (including a huge increase in the availability and power of technology) with yesterday's tools (our caveman brain). When the pressures of modern life meet the ancient circuitry of our brains, anxiety happens. I call this 'the perfect storm', except there's nothing perfect about it.

In our caveman days, our brains convinced us that we were weaker and slower than our predators in an effort to protect us; today, our brains still gauge our social and personal worth based on how we feel we stack up against others. As a result, we constantly make comparisons between ourselves and those around us across a variety of domains, like attractiveness, wealth, intelligence and success. This is 'Social Comparison Theory.'[40]

With the advent and almost universal use of social media, people have even more ways to compare themselves to others, 24 hours a day. All of this makes for an awful lot of pressure on a daily basis. Constant exposure to what everyone else is doing can make us hyper-aware of what we're not doing, which in turn can lead to FOMO (fear of missing out), particularly for younger people. Add to that the constant stream of everyone else's 'highlight reels' (i.e. the best bits of their lives that people choose to portray on social media), and it's easy to feel like you don't quite measure up. If that's so often true for us adults, imagine how your developing and impressionable child might feel!

Once children reach middle childhood they develop an increased awareness of the world beyond their family and close friends. This is when the pressures of comparing themselves to others and conforming to peers becomes apparent. In addition, children now realise that their performance in school must really matter, and *that's* why the grown-ups keep harping on about it …

It's also around this stage in a child's development that bullying can become an inescapable problem, which relates to how children judge themselves against others. Bullying has been around forever, but it's now relentless because of social media. Where once a bullied child got to recover in the evening at home with their family, now the bullying follows them online after school; they can carry it around in their pocket and check in at any time. Whilst there are many advantages to the advent of the smartphone and social media, for children, especially those prone to anxiety, being 'on' all the time keeps their Threat system on high alert, which takes away from their precious downtime.

The burden of great expectations

Dr Colman Noctor, a child and adolescent psychotherapist, puts it this way[41]:

Happiness = Expectations – Reality[42]

With a constant stream of the 'best bits' of everyone else's lives in our pockets – best hair days, school reports, amazing holidays, you name it – we now live in a world that drives our expectations up, up, up. As a result, we've ended up with a situation in which our expectations often far exceed our capacity to meet them.

Children often have high expectations for themselves based on both internal and external pressures – expectations that don't look all that unlike our own: 'If I win, then I'll be happy'; 'If I can look this way, then I'll be happy.'

If children were rewarded more for showing kindness to themselves and others, they'd be much happier and less anxious. They wouldn't care as much about getting medals or the newest haircut. They wouldn't be struggling for the impossible. Instead they'd be encouraged to look inside and find something with much greater meaning.

> It's up to us, step by step and little by little, to go back to the basics of the more important things in life if we feel that external pressures are significantly impacting on our kids. Naturally, we live in the society that we live in, and our power to change it is limited. But the culture that we create within our homes and within our schools is one that we *can* have a real influence over.

Managing our own expectations of our children is an important part of helping them to manage their expectations, as is trying not to live our lives through them – although this is easier said than done. Children have a right to make their own mistakes and to follow their own paths. Remember that supporting them unconditionally through the jungle of life is something they won't get from anyone else. You are their everything in this regard, even though that may be hard to believe sometimes, especially if you're the parent of a teenager!

Doing it for the kids:
checking our motivations as parents

Your role as your child's support system is absolutely crucial. When pressure is coming from everywhere else, you're their stable base; you can remind them who they really are, and what *really* matters.

Having gone through the ups and downs of life yourself, you also have gained perspective, but you must exercise it with caution. Helping your child to realise that their feelings and thoughts are transient, and that there is light at the end of the dark tunnel is one good use of this skill. Nagging children excessively about studying or talking them into doing an activity everyone else is doing is not as good, because it's not necessarily in their best interest.

It's good to encourage children and show them how much you believe in them and in their ability to follow their own star.

But first, remember to ask yourself: 'Am I doing this for me, for someone else or for them?' If it's mostly for them, then you're onto a winner.

If your child is feeling anxious about their performance in something, talking about the equation

Happiness = Expectations – Reality

together might help them to see that their expectations can be very different to what reality brings them. Many things are simply not within our control, so helping anxious kids to see that can be really helpful.

You could also give them an example of a difficulty you encountered as a young person and what that was like for you. Normalising their struggles makes them feel less alone.

Disappointment and not getting what we want are part and parcel of being human, and children need practice in how to manage their hurt feelings, with us standing by their side. We are all human at the end of the day, and resilience comes from facing threats and being able to bounce back with the support of a loved one.

• •

A case in point: Mary

A teenage client, Mary, was taking some important exams. Her father asked me whether he should be urging her to revise at every opportunity. I knew his daughter was quite stressed already and would almost certainly do herself justice in her exams. I was also aware that her school had a huge focus on achieving high marks. So this is what I said to him:

> 'I think Mary is under a huge amount of pressure already. She really wants to do well in her exams and is doing the best that she can. Every time she goes into school, all she hears is "Exams, exams, exams," and "You'll never get another chance."
>
> 'What you can do at home to most nurture Mary is to feed her good brain food and to make sure she gets enough rest and takes breaks between periods of studying. You can also encourage her to do something she enjoys. Help her to get some exercise to refresh her brain, and agree on how much screen time she's getting. Ask her if there's anything more you can do to support her. Be there for her, but try not to add more pressure. Try just to get back to the basics of parenting: love, food, sleep, play.'

Mary's father was relieved by my advice that he didn't have to push his daughter along and that he could focus more on her practical and emotional needs. I also asked him to monitor whether she was experiencing a 'normal' amount of stress or whether her revision seemed to be tipping over into overload, in which case she had the option to come back to see me or for me to visit her at home for a cuppa.

You might be thinking this is all well and good if a child like Mary is focused enough to study, but it's useful to consider what if a child was not so motivated to study, or if something else was going on? In such situations, what is a parent's added pressure going to achieve? Young people have so much going on inside their heads already (e.g. 'Will I get a job?'; 'Will I manage on my own?'; 'Will I make them proud?') that going home should be their respite away from all the noise.

Mary ended up doing well enough in her exams that she could move on to the next level, but most importantly she maintained her mental health as she navigated this life challenge. This also provided another perfect 'survive-and-thrive' moment for her father, who gauged the difficulty, sought help and supported Mary with love and solidarity.

• •

Exams don't measure your true intelligence, creativity and future success, and are not a measure of you as a human being. They are part of the 'game' of life that you have to get through, and then you have your whole life to figure out what your passion is and to carve out your own path.[43]

3
Parents

Dismissing anxious children

Being a child or teenager is even harder than it used to be. Not only is their body changing, their hormones raging, their reasoning brain still developing, but children of all ages are particularly susceptible to peer pressure and comparing themselves negatively to others. In our times, this is made far worse by 24/7 social media. Add to that the pressure to perform in exams and the possibility of trouble at home or school, and you have the perfect recipe for anxiety.

It's easy to dismiss someone who is upset or anxious as being delicate, or as seeking special treatment – a snowflake, as they've come to be known. Calling a child a schoolflake for not going to school is similarly stigmatising, and misses out on the often real difficulties the child may be facing. Here is an example from a newspaper article on the subject of schoolflakes not going to school entitled 'Schoolflakes? The children not going to school … because they don't like it'.

Avoiding school can help an anxious teenager avoid negative emotions associated with school, interaction with peers or teachers, or even tests, if they feel they might not be able to perform well. School refusal can also be a way of gaining attention or support from others and it can provide a way of getting time away from school, thus allowing the adolescent to engage in an activity like

gaming … Parents have reported that when they tell a
teenager he or she can stay home as a result of their
anxiety about school, the child 'immediately cheers up
and becomes significantly less anxious'.[44]

Dismissing children as schoolflakes is not particularly helpful
in trying to help a child with anxiety. First, the label could
make a child feel that they're to blame. Second, it could make
a child resist sharing how they feel. Finally, the label may
discourage parents and school staff from looking beyond the
refusal to go to school to find out exactly what is going on for
the child.

Yes, children sometimes skip school, but the context is the
key to understanding what's motivating it. Questions worth
asking might include: 'Have there been other changes in their
mood or behaviour?' 'What is it about school they may be
avoiding?' 'What is it about home that they feel they need to
be there for?'

This is not to say that we should wrap our children in cotton
wool, wallow in their misery or allow a pattern of school
avoidance to develop. Rather, we need to focus on *acknowledging* any anxious feelings and work together to address any
problems that there might be. By meeting with teachers,
school counsellors and other professionals, parents can work
with others involved in the child's school day to create an overall plan of support if needed, so that the child doesn't miss out
on their education and the crucial social opportunities
provided by going to school.

> Rather than branding today's kids as lacking resilience,
> should we not encourage them to grow it?

Children nowadays may lack resilience compared with those of previous generations, but we need to look at the greater picture of why that might be. Have parents gone overboard by trying to protect their kids from hardship to compensate for something they may have missed out on when they were young?

> Increasingly it seems to me our adolescents and young
> adults are struggling to cope with relatively simple life
> challenges. Has an overly indulgent, softly, softly approach
> left our kids short-changed in terms of resilience and grit?
> Would giving them small challenges to overcome when
> they were younger maybe have helped?[45]

Certainly something to think about. Notwithstanding, labels such as snowflake or schoolflake strengthen stigma, and stigma strengthens silence, particularly when it comes to mental health. For some children who don't even feel deserving of help, these labels encapsulate a reductionist and simplistic view that could further increase the distance between their anxiety and the help they truly deserve. We'll be dealing with the idea of resilience and how to build it later in this chapter and throughout the book.

Before you can help your child, you need to help yourself: anxious parents

One of the questions I inevitably ask parents of anxious children is: 'Does your child remind you of anyone you know?' The answer is fairly predictable.

Many anxious children I've worked with have a parent or caregiver who also struggles with anxiety. Whilst genes and temperament can predispose a child to becoming anxious, parental responses play a role in how their temperament develops over time. Up to 15 per cent of children are born with a temperament that is very reactive to anything new or un-familiar. Children with a reactive temperament are more likely to develop anxiety if their parents over-protect them by letting them avoid things they are afraid of. Children with an anxious temperament need challenges which are 'just right', not too easy and not too tough, which will increase their belief in their ability to cope with a manageable amount of stress with support from their caregivers.

Being a worrier and an overcontroller tends to run in fami-lies. Anxious parents are more likely to have anxious children, and vice versa. Having an anxious child can make a parent more anxious. If you have a tendency towards anxiety, you may not realise how much you actually have in common with your anxious child.

I once asked a parents' group I ran how having an anxious child made them feel. They answered: 'stressed; drained; frus-trated; on edge; on red alert; pent up; trying to stay calm; upset; questioning my parenting; wondering what I'm doing wrong; anxious; tearful; worried for my child'.

When these same parents were asked how their children's anxiety manifested, they said that the children were: 'expecting the worst; obsessing with what might happen; angry; lashing out; panicked; destroying imperfect work; fearing failure; very self-critical; avoiding school; having tummy aches; being indeci-sive; feeling they had the world on their shoulders; having diffi-culty in standing up for themselves; reluctant to join in socially'.

What I found interesting about this exercise was how many similarities there were between the two lists. On the one hand, you can see how anxiety can be reinforced in daily child–parent interactions. On the other, the parent can at least relate to how their child is feeling.

As a result of this connection, one of the best ways of helping a child with anxiety is to reach them through their parents. The parents of anxious children are generally very eager to learn new strategies to help their kids, which is a really positive first step. My role is to take in parents' concerns and challenges, and to try to contain the situation for them. Then it's a case of trying to reduce parents' expectations of getting straight to problem-solving mode – because that's not the most helpful response to begin with. In containing parental concerns and showing compassion for how challenging their situation is, we build a good foundation of safety and connection, from which problem-solving can then evolve.

Anxiety made simple

Question: Where does anxiety come from?

Answer: Anxiety comes from a part of the brain called the amygdala. It's designed to help us survive attack, and it switches on when it thinks you're in danger. It's not very big, looks like an almond and sits at the back of each of your ears, and is always scanning for trouble. Some call it a 'fierce warrior' because it always has your back and is incredibly hardworking.

If your amygdala spots trouble, it immediately gives your body what it needs to be strong, fast and powerful. It floods your body with oxygen and hormones like adrenaline, which your body can use as fuel to power your muscles to attack (fight), run away (flight) or shut down (freeze).

If the threat isn't real and you don't need to fight for your life, run away or shut down, then there's nothing to burn up all that fuel that has flooded your body. The tension builds and builds – and that's why you feel as rotten as you do when you have anxiety.

The amygdala switches on when it thinks there might be trouble, but it thinks lots of things mean trouble.

Apart from the fight-flight-freeze response, the amygdala also switches on worried thoughts; these are built into your system to keep you alert and to protect you from danger. Fear of separation from someone you love, worrying about something bad happening, feeling not good enough, excluded, lonely or rejected, even embarrassment – all count as 'trouble', so you can see how the amygdala can go into overdrive easily enough!

Many parents I see are what I would call mildly anxious. However, trouble can arise when a parent's own anxiety reaches a problematic level. Because children's anxiety is very sensitive to caregivers' responses, an anxious parent may inadvertently play a role in maintaining a child's anxiety. When this happens, it's hard for the child or the parent to see where the cycle of stress between them begins or ends.

There are several ways in which parental responses can be problematic. Because children naturally look to their parents for information and guidance on how to interpret their worlds and their emotions, if they sense their parent becoming anxious (e.g. through their words, actions or reactions), then this could well magnify their own feelings.

If a parent starts to take on their child's worries themselves, then the child can believe that they were right to feel anxious in the first place, and that there is indeed a threat. On the other hand, if a parent dismisses the child's worries – telling them to 'get over it' or to 'grow a thick skin' – the child may end up feeling that they were wrong to be anxious, that they can't trust their feelings or that there's something wrong with them.

These responses are more common than you might think. You may have used both strategies in the heat of an anxious moment or in the absence of knowing what to do:

> If a child is worried about going to school, a parent might initially listen and worry with them [strategy 1] before getting exasperated and angry, trying to force the child out the door, which leads to a meltdown [strategy 2]. These negative cycles leave everyone feeling bad and are damaging if repeated daily.[46]

To break the pattern of reacting unhelpfully to an anxious child, the most important thing to do is to pause for a moment when your child becomes anxious and to commit to remaining calm and still. You're aiming to counterbalance their heightened state. If it helps, visualise yourself as a still point (like an anchor), even though your child may be in a whirlwind out at sea. This is easier said than done, especially if you're prone to worry yourself, so there may be an element of faking the calm to begin with.[47]

The next step is to respond warmly and empathetically to your child, and to try to understand and acknowledge the source of their worry. Both 'Anchoring' and helping a child to 'Feel felt' are covered in the SAFE Chain of Resilience on page 77.

Managing these early relationships and the origins of stress in young people were at the forefront of my mind when I became involved in an RTÉ 1 documentary called *Stressed* (see page 279, note 9). In addition to introducing a baby mental health poster campaign to parents at a local clinic, it also featured an adult volunteer who was seeing me for counselling. In speaking to parents about the origins of stress, our aim was to show how everyday parenting moments from the very earliest days and throughout a child's life provide us with precious opportunities to build connection and strengthen our children's resilience. I really enjoyed my experience of meeting and working with Jonathan.

• •

A case in point: Jonathan

Jonathan had contacted the programme as he was struggling with the stress of his busy work life and felt unable to step off the 'hamster wheel', with all of its daily demands. He desperately wanted advice on how to rebalance his life to enjoy more quality time with his family and to live more in the moment, rather than feeling constantly overwhelmed.

At the time, compassion-focused therapy was becoming increasingly important as one of the most effective stress-beating strategies, and so a compassionate approach was what I felt would best meet Jonathan's needs. Despite our relatively short time together over nine sessions, my hope was that developing his ability to be compassionate to himself would offer more than a quick fix, coupled with us looking at the deeper emotional patterns that had led to him feeling stressed.

After an in-depth discussion about his daily life and what he was hoping to gain from the sessions, I explained about the Three Circles and asked him to draw his Drive, Threat and Soothing circles to scale and show the interaction between them.

Jonathan drew his Drive circle the largest, his Threat circle smaller and his Soothing circle much smaller still. We also drew an arrow from Threat to Drive, as it was clear that something powerful was feeding his overactive Drive, which is common for people experiencing high levels of stress.

Drawing his Three Circles made Jonathan think twice about the way he was just going, going, going all the time (Threat feeding Drive), without giving enough time or energy to nurturing himself or his relationships (Soothing). It was no wonder that he was running himself into the ground.

At some point in his early life, Jonathan started to believe that continuously pushing himself harder and harder was the key to his happiness. When he was older, this developed into the idea that 'Once I have X amount of money and success, then my family will be comfortable and I'll be happy.'

When Jonathan pushed himself too hard, he felt understandably depleted and unable to engage as much with his family. His family time was what he most valued, and it was what nurtured him. Without the security he gained from a close relationship with his family, he found himself unable to appreciate his achievements along the way. He was always under pressure, and felt he was chasing happiness. His defence mechanism was to switch off his emotions to cope with his experience of family breakdown when he was a child, so the challenge was for him to learn to feel all his feelings and yet still be driven and feel like himself.

Jonathan was very open to engaging in therapy and embraced the opportunity for reflection, which he said could not have come at a better time. He was surprised that what started out as thinking he would gain a few techniques to manage his stress ended up as something much deeper, delving into why he felt like he felt, and how to use self-kindness and mindfulness exercises. We explored how his overactive Drive may have affected both his behaviour and others' feelings towards him, and, although this was understandably difficult, he was open to learning more.

By the time we had finished our sessions, we had become so immersed in the therapeutic work that the documentary almost seemed like an afterthought. None of our therapy had been filmed, except for one final shot where I asked him to redraw his

Three Circles as he now saw them to give the audience a flavour of CFT: Drive was a bit smaller, Threat much smaller, and his Soothing circle had grown significantly since we'd begun. We also noticed that his Drive circle was being fed by Soothing instead of Threat which was a welcome change.

Jonathan's progress showed, too, in his new daily routine. He left work earlier, spent more time with his family, started to be on time and paused more to look at the world around him. He was beginning to explore his feelings, which had been relatively unchartered territory for him up to now. Jonathan had been afraid that focusing on his Soothing system might make him complacent or lazy, but that was not how it panned out. He was driven *and* nurtured at the same time, without stress taking over his life. In his own powerful words, 'I want to live life to the full and not work to live.'

....

Many parents feel like Jonathan to some degree; we're all trying so damn hard to do the best that we can in so many different areas of our lives, it's nearly impossible to keep up – unless we ground ourselves with compassion and support.

The problem is that, like Jonathan, many parents I see don't engage in many daily activities which fall into the Soothing circle, giving them the support they need and replenishing their batteries. If this can be traced back to their not being soothed enough or treated with compassion as a child, they may not know how to calm and nurture themselves as adults. In adults, not being able to self-soothe leads to ignoring signs of significant stress, and not seeking much-needed help or social support, which has knock on effects on the parent's ability to soothe their child.

Parental transmission of anxiety:
helicopter parenting

As I now observe my parents as grandparents, I can see how their anxieties became my anxieties as a child. Their bubble-wrap and overprotective style of parenting left me unable to explore life without extreme caution. Being a bubble-wrapped child has made me a very anxious adult.

A parent who pays extremely close attention to their child and overprotects them is increasingly known as a 'helicopter parent'. I'm not a big fan of the term, as it blames a parent who has developed this strategy for very good reason, whether due to a childhood wound, a later trauma or the impact of our fear-driven world.

Parents who are overprotective are often anxious themselves and feel a strong urge to control situations. They may do this because they fear losing control, which could stem from earlier traumatic events that left them feeling helpless and vulnerable. They may feel they need to be there for their kids 24/7, perhaps as a way of righting a wrong from their earlier lives – say, if their own parents weren't around enough for them when they most needed them.

Anxiety made simple

Question: How is the amygdala like a smoke alarm?

Answer: When we feel a lot of anxiety, the amygdala's alarm system acts like a wonky smoke alarm that goes off every time you (barely) burn your toast in the morning. An alarm system is brilliant if you need to save yourself from a real fire, but not so brilliant if it can't tell the difference between smoke from a fire and a little bit of smoke from burnt toast!

Alongside other parts of the brain, the amygdala is also in charge of memories, which means that if something you experience now feels in any way similar to something you found frightening in the past, then it can bring up negative memories, feelings and images.

For example, if you've had a prior bad experience swimming in water before, your amygdala will sound the alarm if you go anywhere near water and get you ready to protect yourself without there actually being a current threat. The awful feeling in your gut will make you think that all water must be scary and will stop you going near it, but it's actually your amygdala hijacking the logical part of your brain, the prefrontal cortex. That's the part that usually helps you to calm down; it's where your reasoning and problem-solving take place.

Like a smoke alarm, anxiety is helpful when it works correctly, like when there is a real threat, or when you just need that bit of get-up-and-go to do well at something. For example, a healthy dose of nerves can be useful to help you perform well in an exam, but too many can feel overwhelming.

Some call the brain's smoke alarm an 'amygdala hijack', because the amygdala is the boss of scary situations and hijacks the rest of the brain – unless you know how to calm it.

Anxiety becomes a problem when our body reacts as if it's in real danger when in reality there is no danger. If this happens often enough, it can affect your home or school life and how you feel about yourself. That's when you know you need to talk to someone about how you feel, so you can get some help and support; the same is true if you notice this in your child.

• •

A case in point: me

Having kids is a real challenge if you have a tendency towards controlling situations. Kids can be loud, unpredictable, messy and unaware of danger, while having a natural developmental need to explore their environments and master new things. All of which is tough for a parent for whom being in control feels safer and more containable.

I know the feeling. My alarm bells ring loud and clear every time my girls face potential dangers, like a busy car park or a high climbing frame. I know that my fight-flight-freeze response goes off without much provocation, and that my danger detector is way too sensitive. Even hearing a fight brewing between them is enough to send me into emotional overdrive.

What I have come to realise over the years is that I'm what some would call a bit of a control freak. I may have been born that way, but I certainly experienced my fair share of anxiety when I was younger, and people used to say of me as a child that I was overly conscientious in a way that was much beyond my years. That was a heavy weight to carry, believe you me.

My transition to parenthood was pretty hard. I suddenly realised that I had to look after another human being, and it terrified the life out of me. How could I possibly manage to keep my child safe and happy throughout her life? More importantly, how would I achieve it with the level of control I was used to having in other parts of my life? Impossible!

Once I had our second child, and as the girls grew older, I realised there was no such thing as perfect and that I couldn't control everything. I came to see that my rigidity was preventing me being fully present and available to them. I have a very playful side too, but when it came to bedtime, for instance, I would feel a huge pressure to ensure that they got into bed on time, by hook or by crook. It wasn't a pretty sight!

I used to hate it when the children got out of bed after I had tucked them in – it was as if by getting up they were proving that I'd lost control of the situation. So I'd be listening out for the slightest noise, and if I heard anything I'd shoot straight up the stairs to see what was the matter.

One evening my husband asked me, 'Do you ever need time to settle after you go to bed or go to the toilet or whatever?'

'Yeah, sometimes I do.'

The girls also needed their time to settle before sleep, and would call down to us if they needed help. Maybe, suggested my husband, I should leave them to settle for a few minutes and not rush up at every sound. This would also teach them a valuable lesson in settling themselves.

He was right. Yes, it was hard to stop myself from reacting immediately, but I realised I had a choice. It's in these small moments that parents can pause, and take a step back from their default control patterns. I'm lucky to have someone with a calm presence who reins me back in when I need a reality check. Getting support from someone you trust can be really helpful in giving you some perspective on anxiety. I still fluctuate between being too controlling and not controlling enough, but I'm trying not to sweat the small stuff and now work on being 'good enough'.

....

For parents of anxious children, being overprotective or trying to be indispensable is reinforced when your child doesn't *want* to get any distance from you because they want protection from whatever is making them anxious. This can make it even more difficult for parents to change their responses to the anxiety. For example, many parents in such situations rarely take time for themselves as a couple or even on their own. This is totally understandable, as the last thing you want to do is to provoke a meltdown by planning to go out: 'How can you go out,' you can imagine your child saying, 'when you should be here with me to keep me safe?' It can seem easier to just stay at home, can't it? But is this simply a case of short-term gain for long-term pain? Could your attempt to avoid a confrontation itself be feeding into your child's anxiety? If we stay at home all the time, are we teaching our children that they're right to be worried, that there is indeed a good reason to be fearful? Or could we be sending them the message that we don't trust in their ability to manage without us?

It can help to think about the differences between the intended and unintended consequences of what we do. What we hope to achieve in a situation is an intended consequence; less desirable outcomes are called unintended consequences.

In the case of being indispensable to a child, intended consequences may include keeping them safe, calming them down and feeling in control. There can be unintended consequences too, such as reinforcing the child's anxious thoughts and behaviours, and preventing them from trying something new or learning to cope for themselves. Consider as well the unintended consequences of not giving yourself some time to yourself as a parent. How can you begin to help your child to fill their cup if yours is almost empty?

Naturally your child still needs you to be their secure base when confronting tough situations, but being an anchor is that bit different for an anxious child, as it requires a more finely tuned balance of holding tight and letting go than might be the case for another child. In empowering children, we need to find the balance between being an overprotective, indispensable parent and being over-permissive or letting them face their demons alone. In the long term, we want to prepare them to make their own decisions and equip them with the skills for managing the unexpected.

Although you're in charge of many parts of your child's life, it's helpful to know that you can't control their anxious behaviour. You can try to cultivate a relaxed environment in which all feelings, good and bad, are welcomed and where they're more likely to display positive, worry-free behaviour, but at the end of the day kids are unpredictable little beings with their own minds and wants and needs.

Controlling *your response* to your child's behaviour is the only thing you have control over. So increasing your own self-awareness and your capacity to reflect and respond to your children's needs is where we're going next.

The power of reflection

Making sense of your life is the best gift you can give your child.

How you reflect on yourself as a parent and make sense of your childhood experiences has a profound impact on how you parent your child. A parent's capacity for understanding and reflecting on their own thoughts, feelings, behaviour and intentions, as well as those of their child, is crucial in nurturing the quality of the child–parent attachment bond.

As parents, growing and understanding ourselves frees up our emotional space so we are better able to interpret and respond to our children's needs. For example, during a really difficult moment, if I am aware that my child isn't intentionally trying to push my buttons, and can consider that their behaviour may be due to them being tired or lonely, then I'm more likely to respond to them in a more understanding and calm way.

'Reflective parenting'[48] describes a parent tuning in to their child's internal state, which paves the way for the child to understand themselves and recognise their desires, feelings, thoughts and wishes as valid and separate from those of their parents. A reflective parent tries to:

- hold their child in mind
- tune in to their child's thoughts and feelings
- tune in to their own thoughts and feelings
- understand that their own and their child's thoughts and feelings are intertwined
- realise the separation between their child's thoughts and feelings and their own
- stand back and recognise what they are doing and not doing to meet the child's needs
- let their child know that they are understood using both verbal and non-verbal gestures
- make a balanced choice in the child's best interest.

Granted it's a long list, but it's one that can be improved on bit by bit if we take some time to focus on the way we were parented and how this may be impacting on our own parenting:

> Contrary to what many people believe, your early experiences do not determine your fate. If you had a difficult childhood but have come to make sense of those experiences, you are not bound to re-create the same negative interactions with your own children. Without such self-understanding, science has shown that history will repeat itself, as negative patterns of family interactions are passed down through the generations.[49]

A research study I keep going back to found that even when parents had experienced high levels of stress as children, it was their degree of reflection which was the best predictor of a secure attachment with their child.[50] So if a parent grows up with many stressors in their lives, it is their ability to stand back and notice the impact on themselves and their parenting which plays a deciding role in how they will attune to their children's needs:

> More important for our children than merely what
> happened to us in the past is the way we have come to
> process and understand it. The opportunity to change and
> grow continues to be available throughout our lives.[51]

This information can bring a lot of hope to parents who have had difficult childhoods. It has the power to change the way they relate to their children, creating newer, healthier relationship patterns, which are likely to be passed down from generation to generation. Pretty amazing isn't it?

Fortunately, even if a parent hasn't experienced a secure attachment as a child, there is the possibility of 'earned security', which is done through forming secure relationships later in life and making sense of how childhood experiences impact us and our parenting.

The good news is that not only can security be learnt, but that a parent's reflection skills can be improved, if we invest time in looking after ourselves as parents. Prioritising self-care is vital in building our capacity for reflection and our emotional reserves to equip us for the job of parenting. The fact is that we can't meet our children's needs or fill their emotional cups unless we fill ours first. If we're OK, they're OK. Simple as.

No one is saying any of this is easy. It can be hard to look into your past and remember how your own needs were met or unmet by your parents. But it's worth the effort as over time the awareness will enable you to make calmer choices about how you respond to your child, with positive ripples resonating far beyond your relationship.

Tuning in to your shark music

This brings me to a gem of a concept I encountered in my training as a Circle of Security™ parenting programme facilitator, where echoes of the way we were parented as children are referred to as 'shark music'.[52] This concept originally came from a parent who said that having to respond to their child's needs sometimes made them panic and experience a strong flood of emotion, just like when they heard the menacing soundtrack from the film *Jaws*. This struck a chord with other parents and forms the basis for the following visual exercise which I show to parents attending the parenting programme.

In the first video clip parents are shown someone walking down a path through a forest, turning a corner and encountering a beach at the bottom. Beautiful classical music plays in the background. Parents are then asked how they felt after watching it. Answers varied from 'relaxed' to 'excited' to 'peaceful'. There was definitely a sense of positive anticipation for what lay ahead; people wanted to explore.

The second clip showed exactly the same forest path, the same corner and the same beach at the bottom of the path – but this time with the crescendo of the infamous *Jaws* music playing in the background. Asked how they felt after the second clip, their answers ranged from 'scared' to 'terrified' to 'panicked'. Their positive anticipation had turned into absolute dread of what lay ahead.

This exercise was used to illustrate how our past experiences often feature as the background music that shapes how we respond to our children. As a result of these experiences, parents are more comfortable with some of their children's needs than others. When parents hear that shark music, it can have more to do with their own childhood than with whatever threat their children might be facing, which interferes with their ability to contain their children's emotions when needed or to foster independence when needed.

For example, one of your own parents may have been comfortable with you climbing to the top of a climbing frame, while the other may have gone into an absolute tizzy that you would fall. So, you would have learned to express your need to explore and climb in front of one parent, but would have hidden it from the other.

But how did one of your parent's internal alarm systems develop to ring so loudly while the other was so comfortable with you taking risks? Consider too what their reactions would have been if you had fallen: one might have been more hugs and kisses if you fell, the other more 'Get up now – no blood, you're fine.'

The truth is that children learn to be sensitive to all of this from their early experiences with their parents. Given that parents are their child's secure base from birth, children will naturally look to them for information and guidance on how to interpret their worlds.

Every time a parent says something, does something or reacts to something, their child is observing and learning from their behaviour. Just like me, you must often experience these copycat 'mini you' moments of your children mimicking you in some little way. Most of the time it's endearing, but sometimes it can be a bit worrying.

For example, when I bring my girls to the pool I've heard them look around and say, 'Thank God it's not busy today, Mum! It was horrible here the last time when it was so packed and loud. Hopefully it will be nice and quiet today.' Was this what they really thought? I very much doubt it. My children repeated what I'd said the previous time because they had learned that I heard my shark music in an overcrowded pool.

Children are always on the lookout for their parents' moods and emotional availability, which we often reveal without even knowing it. More than once, my eldest daughter has met me first thing in the morning, inspected me with laser eyes and commented, 'Great mummy, you're in a good mood'. Equally, she scans for when I'm emotionally drained which is when she bypasses me entirely in favour of her daddy! Smart girlie.

Because children can change their behaviour to match your mood, it can make it difficult for parents to recognise or to respond differently to our children's needs.

> The brain continually prepares itself for the future based on what has previously happened, and these past experiences strongly influence how we understand what we see and feel in the present. We all parent in a particular way due to a combination of our past experiences and the choices we make in the present. Learning from our past experiences is a good thing, but it can also act as a buried land mine which limits us from recognising our own shark music and responding sensitively to our children's needs.
>
> When we have had scary past experiences, as many parents have, our shark music also makes us afraid or uncomfortable with feelings that are actually safe. When our shark music limits our ability to respond to our children's feelings, children learn to hide or feel ashamed of them. This is a big problem, because we're teaching them to fear emotions that are actually safe, healthy and essential in life.

What to do? The choice before you is that you can protect yourself from further pain by avoiding their need or you can respond to your child's need in spite of the discomfort it causes you.

The good news is that by calling shark music out for what it is, and reflecting on what our children need in the moment, we can actually turn the music down. Exploring our history of negative experiences enables us to better respond to our child's actual current situation and to be with them in it. Tuning in to your shark music – the things that make you anxious – could be something you do on your own, but many parents need support, be that a good friend or seeing a professional. Either way, what you're looking to do is:[53]

- Recognise the anxiety when it comes: 'Ah, there's my shark music again.'
- Honour the anxiety: 'I'm hurting now because my child's particular need is triggering my shark music.'
- Respond to your child's need: 'I'll make a conscious effort to respond differently.'

This last step is hard, so let me give you an example. When my children used to come to me with a skinned knee, I found it really difficult to comfort them. It was like a part of me froze and I couldn't fully empathise. This is still a hard thing for me to admit.

Now that I know about shark music, I can see that I developed this response because that is how some of my minor physical hurts may have been dealt with as a child. By no means is this a blame game; shark music helps us to see why we respond in certain ways and recognise how these patterns repeat themselves across generations.

This is where building our ability to reflect is so crucial. We all struggle, but now that I know that I struggle with this particular need from my children I don't blame myself, because I didn't know any better. I didn't know why I was reacting in a cold way, so it was hard to show myself any compassion – or to be compassionate towards my children. As Maya Angelou once wrote, 'I did what I knew how to do. Now that I know better, I do better.'

Changing my automatic response hasn't been easy. Sometimes you just have to fake it till you make it, and that's what I had to do. Now when one of my daughters hurts herself and looks to me for comfort, although I feel that iciness and anxiety inside myself, I try hard to focus on her need for comfort and to be with her in the moment. It's hard, but it's been pretty healing too:

> Understanding your shark music's origins has a way of easing your stress and boosting your self-compassion along with compassion for your child. You can definitely turn the volume down.[54]

Resilience: the paradoxical gift of pain

If we let ourselves feel it, we give ourselves a better chance to heal it. From the moment we have kids we're all full of the best intentions, and we're hardwired to try to protect them from harm. But protecting them from harm is one thing – protecting them from everything is quite another. Are we really helping children if we shield them from the everyday challenges – and let's face it, everyday pain – of being human?

To develop resilience, a child needs a secure relationship with their parent, secure enough to learn how to face a threat that they feel they can manage. As adults, we realise that what a child finds threatening – sitting at a new table at school, going to a birthday party, learning to swim, trying new foods or doing tests at school – usually feels manageable to us. But part of learning not to dismiss your child's worries is coming to understand that what looks like a small threat to us may seem very unmanageable to them. All things are relative. So, we listen, we accept that they're dealing with big feelings like fear, anger or sadness, and we go from there.

What a parent can do to help their child with these big feelings is to lead by example. We all make mistakes, we all have tough moments, we all feel pain and suffering. If your child sees you accept and confront all these feelings as they come, they'll know it's possible.

We can teach our children how to be human in an imperfect world, a world where things can and do go wrong, a world where we're 'filled with confusing needs and uncomfortable emotions, hapless and flawed, stumbling about in an ever-learning state of glorious imperfection'.[55]

Naturally, parents still hold the responsibility to be the bigger and wiser ones when responding to their children's big feelings. But recognising your children as being their own little people and acknowledging your shared humanity seems to take the pressure off a bit.

> It helps to see your child as a little person rather than
> 'your' child who 'ought' to behave in a particular way.
> When things go wrong, which they inevitably do, it can
> be a relief to say, 'You're human, I'm human, this isn't
> working, how can we get through this together?'[56]

One way of parenting your child without so much fear is to show that you, too, are human.

> Your kids are constantly on the lookout for how *you* manage tough situations.

Part of a secure child–parent relationship is the importance of a parent modelling self-compassion. Do you show yourself kindness, or are you very critical of yourself? Do you push your feelings down for fear of them overwhelming you, or do you accept your thoughts and feelings as they come?

We all have things we can improve on in how we respond to our kids, but the way we relate to ourselves during tough moments has a lasting impact on them and will often play out in how they relate to themselves. If a child sees their parent beating themselves up for something, the message that sends will be stronger than anything the parent says.

On the other hand, if children witness their parents embracing what it means to be human, being kind and gentle with themselves, and being able to apologise and to forgive following inevitable mistakes and misunderstandings, then this will give them a solid foundation for compassionately regulating their emotions and caring for themselves.

When kids who are struggling practise self-compassion, powerful things happen: their sense of self-worth, resilience and ability to cope with problems improve in all settings.[57]

Sitting with your feelings – including pain

Pain is part of life; ordinary, irritating pain, like minor disappointments or embarrassment, all the way up to major traumas, losses, separation and bereavements.

Our relationship with pain is hugely important, as is how we choose to respond to our own and our children's painful moments. Many parents I've met have real difficulty in 'sitting with' painful feelings, be these their own or their children's, for very understandable reasons relating to their own childhood histories.

In order to help our children, we need to come to terms with all our feelings. Sitting with your feelings means noticing how you feel – and *just feeling that way* without berating yourself for it, even if it's painful or upsetting.

• •

A case in point: James

James, the single father of a seven-year-old, bravely shared with me the fact that he was afraid of his son's big feelings as a result of his own feelings having been 'frozen' as a child. Because his father wasn't around, and his mother struggled with her mental health, James, as the eldest, took on the responsibility for looking after his younger siblings. Although he said his mum had tried her best, and he now felt awfully guilty for having questioned her support, James survived that difficult time by pushing down his feelings of anger, sadness and fear, knowing his mother was probably too overwhelmed or unable to contain his big emotions.

Not only did James learn that he had to try to stifle his painful feelings as there was no one at home to talk to, he was also battling against societal messages such as 'Boys don't cry' and 'Man up and just get on with it.' These are the kinds of messages that harm boys and men of all ages, and are leading to the incredibly high rate of mental ill health and suicide among men that we see today.

Because he had to hide his feelings when he was a child, James became hypersensitive to his own children's emotional pain. To ensure that his own history wouldn't be repeated, he described needing to be one step ahead of what was going on all the time. He was overwhelmed every time his son became upset, since he was working so hard to pre-empt his son's feelings. The pressure he was putting himself under had become too much. 'How will I hold it together enough to help him?' he'd think. Although he tried his hardest to listen to his son, he felt a huge weight of responsibility on his shoulders to try to fix things yet again, just as he had done all throughout his childhood. He also felt a deep sense of protectiveness as a single dad.

'I can't let him sit in fear,' he told me. Meanwhile, James's son was learning to suppress his feelings, leading to explosions of anger and anxiety both at home and at school. By trying to shelter his son from his fear, and being physically and emotionally present for him all the time, as his own mother had not been, James believed that he was protecting his son from the pain he himself had suffered as a child.

It was only as we explored it that James realised that if this pattern were to continue, his son might never learn to develop his own coping skills. James could also see how spreading himself too thinly was impacting on his own emotional well-being, another pattern he was unconsciously repeating from childhood.

This is where the paradoxical gift of pain became clear. Denying his son the full experience of pain was denying him the experience of being human and of learning how to cope. James loved his son more than anything. He said that he wanted to heal for himself and for his son too. Part of their healing would be in the witnessing of pain and the realisation that pain is part of being human. Almost as importantly, pain is also usually a naturally short-lived experience, if only we let it do its thing.

··

'First the pain, then the rising'

The author and activist Glennon Doyle once gave a talk entitled 'First the pain, then the rising',[58] in which she told the story of a mother who felt like a failure because her son was in pain and there was nothing she could do to 'fix' it. 'Every day I look at him and I think, "Oh my God, I have one job. My one job was to protect him from pain, and I couldn't do it," and I feel like such a failure.' When Doyle asked her to pick three words to describe the type of man she was trying to raise, the mother answered: 'I want him to be kind. I want him to be wise. And I want him to be resilient.'

Doyle went on to say:

> What is it in human life that creates kindness and
> wisdom and resilience? It's pain. That's it. It's the struggle.
> It's not having nothing to overcome. It's overcoming and
> overcoming and overcoming. So, is it possible that we are
> trying to protect our children from the one thing that will
> allow them to become the people we dream they'll be? And
> is it possible that we all feel like failures because we have
> the wrong job description? Because it was never our job,
> nor our right, to protect our children from their pain. Our
> job is to point them directly towards it and say, 'Baby, that
> was meant for you and I see your fear, and it's real, and it's
> big, but I see your courage and it's bigger.'

Not everyone will take to Doyle's approach; not everyone will
want to or indeed even be able to see pain in this way. It's a
very tall order for a parent to welcome pain and fear into their
child's life. I wonder, does knowing that there can be a gift in
the pain change anything for you?

This is what compassionate parenting is all about. We don't
necessarily change the pain that we or our children will experience, but we change our *relationship* with the pain – and,
hopefully, theirs. To do this we need to take a step back and
look deep inside at how we deal with painful feelings, which
usually stems from how our feelings were managed when we
were kids.

Being an emotional anchor

We also do this by realising our crucial role as parents in
anchoring our children to safety when they feel overwhelmed
by their feelings. From this point on I'll be using the metaphor
of you being your child's 'emotional anchor'; where they learn

to rely on you as either a secure base from which to support their exploration or as a safe haven into which you'll welcome them back.

When your child feels threatened by their environment or by their anxious thoughts, they're more likely to seek you out as their emotional anchor and less likely to feel inclined to explore their world. While this is a positive sign as it shows their attachment to you as a source of comfort and reassurance, you'll see that there's a fine balance to be reached between holding them safe and encouraging their gradual exposure to the things they fear.

This balance can be challenging and requires a lot of scaffolding for you as a parent. The compassionate approach fits the bill because it acknowledges that all emotions, including anxiety, have a function in communicating to us something important about our inner state and we should use these as signposts to what we most need.

The feeling of anxiety is an emotion that we all experience by simply being a human being. But for some it can just take over and interfere with their ability to function, as they'll be unwilling – and therefore unable – to explore their environment and learn new things. The reasons for this will vary from child to child, but once you gain a clearer understanding of your child's development and circumstances, the origins of their anxiety may begin to become clear.

In guiding you on your path using a compassionate approach, I have developed the four steps of what I call the SAFE Chain of Resilience to support you in navigating your child's anxiety. These steps comprise:

- **S**elf-care: how you look after yourself as a parent and regulate your emotions
- **A**nchoring: how you can help your child feel safe
- **F**eeling felt: how you can help your child feel connected

- **E**mpowerment: how you can empower your child to manage
  their anxiety

These steps will need to be worked on in this particular order
to best tap in to your child's brain development and their inner
resources (see Chapter 6). In this way, the tougher moments
you have been surviving up to now could become precious
opportunities to further strengthen your relationship with
your child, and ultimately help to build their lifelong
resilience.

4
Children

Anxiety feels real

The reality of what anxiety feels like for a child was powerfully illustrated in a letter written by 11-year-old Tommy to his mother:

Without you Mom:
 Sometimes I feel so sad without you Mom
 Sometimes I cry and just can't stop
 Sometimes I hide under my bed where no one can see
 When you go out I feel so lost and scared, like the worst thing in the world is going to happen. I wish you wouldn't leave me anymore
 If you go away much more even to the shop I may as well be dead because I'll feel so alone and so sick. Someone may as well lock me up and throw away the key!
 When I have to leave you to go to school I get terrible pains in my belly. Teachers try to help and say I'll be OK, but I WON'T BE OK, nothing is OK without you Mom!
 What I really want is for you to stay with me forever so I feel safe and not so sick in my belly anymore. I'm tired of feeling alone and afraid all on my own.
 Before you even try to tell me it's OK I want you to know this LOUD AND CLEAR: THIS FEELING IS UNHELPABLE!

PS No one ever listens to me so I am writing this hoping
that you will listen Mom.

So very sad, isn't it, for a little boy to feel so alone in his scary
feelings? Like many other anxious children, Tommy feels
stuck in a cage of anxiety, always looking inwards. He's clutch-
ing onto safety and is too afraid to ask for help or to hope for
better days.

Imagine the hopelessness of your feelings being 'unhelpable', of feeling unheard and misunderstood. Tommy's deep
insecurity every time that his mother went out showed up as
big, messy feelings: tummy aches, bad sleep, avoiding friends
and dreading school. Fortunately, he was not consistently in
such a state of high anxiety, but when it hit, boy did it really
hit.

This scenario may seem extreme to some, but Tommy's
experience might resonate with you in some small way. When
a child expresses an 'unhelpable' feeling, think how overwhelming it is for their parents to hear that. As a parent, you're
meant to know how to make things better for your child; you
have this instinctive urge to protect them, yet you feel powerless in all your efforts. What to do?

Telling you that your child's anxiety feels real, just like
yours, may not be news to you. As we've discussed, many
parents of anxious children may have also experienced anxiety
as children, so the reality of Tommy's worries could feel quite
familiar.

Anxiety made simple

Question: Am I the only one with anxiety?

Answer: Anxiety is common in kids and grown-ups, and affects about one in eight kids in the world. Because of this, there's a good chance that three to four kids in your class will know what you're going through – because they've been through it before, or they're going through it right now. Although lots of people get it, anxiety can feel a bit different for everyone.

Kids of all ages can get anxious for lots of reasons. Sometimes we don't know why, or there may not even be a reason that makes sense to us, and that's OK too. With help from the people who love you, you'll feel better with a bit of time and a bit of practice.

I was once that anxious child myself, so I know what it feels like to have the weight of the world on my shoulders and to feel all alone with my worries, just like Tommy. My biggest fear was getting lost in a big, crowded place, dreading I might never find my parents again, or that they might never find me again, or worse still … what if they didn't even look for me?

The innocence of it, to believe that you won't be found again – but did it ever feel real to me! To the now grown-up part of me, this doesn't make a huge amount of sense, but as a child it was really, really scary. That was just one of my many worries: my brain was like Velcro for anything remotely scary, whether it related to me, my family, friends, or something out in the big bad world.

After another failed trip to the doctor, where 'nothing physically wrong' was found to explain my recurring tummy aches,
I felt like shouting from the rooftops: 'How can you say there's
nothing wrong with me when my tummy is telling me there is
and when I feel like my world is turning upside down?!'

When you suffer from anxiety, children and adults alike lose
the power to trust their own feelings. This makes it hard to
believe that you'll be able to cope. Because so many situations
feel threatening, you end up feeling really confused about
what is safe and what isn't. It's like your brain and body are
telling you big, fat lies, which to a small child feels really
unsettling and lonely. Even if there is no apparent danger, it
starts to feel safer to avoid even mildly challenging situations
altogether than to risk the dread deep inside you that something will go wrong.

Telling a child that a perceived threat is only in their head,
or that there's nothing to worry about, invalidates the child's
feelings and doesn't help at all in that particular moment. Not
only does a child lose trust in their own feelings and in their
ability to cope, but you risk unintentionally sending the
message that the child's body and mind aren't to be trusted.
This message is of course not intentional from a parent's point
of view; they're simply trying to do the right thing by their
child by protecting or distracting them from their negative
feelings.

But the truth is that trying to gloss over anxiety, hoping that
it goes away, will not make it go away.

When a child shows an adult that something is wrong, be it
through words, physical symptoms or behaviour, they're
recruiting us to help them feel safe and less alone. Telling that
anxious child there's nothing to worry about does *not* stop
them worrying. You may have noticed this by now.
Unfortunately, it can also risk making the threat bigger; after
all, the one person they recruited to bring them back to safety

doesn't seem to get it. And that is why anxiety can be a really lonely place to be.

I remember my siblings telling me that the powder the doctor had given me to make my belly feel better was only fake. That stung. I didn't need a placebo powder to make me feel better. In retrospect, maybe what I needed was for an adult to say, 'I can see something doesn't feel right for you' or 'It makes sense that you feel the way you do.' Perhaps we could have made some progress from there.

At the same time, like a lot of children, I was bloody good at hiding my worries. It was my silly belly aches that gave the game away. Looking back, I get why it all happened as it did. I don't at all blame my parents, as there was far less awareness back then and they believed they were doing the best for me.

My parents at that time couldn't have known to link my tummy aches and fear of crowded places to my worries about family, school and moving to another country. Our doctor didn't ask me if anything was the matter, although now that I think about it, I must indeed have been prescribed a placebo because he couldn't find anything wrong. And my teacher didn't know anything was wrong, because I made damn sure I was the good little quiet child, doing my work meticulously and not giving her any bother.

Anxiety wears a lot of disguises. From myriad physical symptoms, to anger and disruptive behaviour, to appearing to be 'just fine', anxiety can be difficult for children and their parents, doctors and teachers to spot. Add to that a parent's distress at seeing their child in pain and their uncertainty about how to respond, and anxiety gets that little bit trickier to see.

Having an anxious child and responding to their daily worries can be exhausting and requires a *lot* of patience. You've got to dig deep, haven't you? To complicate matters, an anxious parent may become overly worried about their child's anxiety, and can manifest this worry either verbally or non-verbally. Logically enough, this makes the child more anxious, as they conclude, 'If my parents are so worried, then there really must be something to worry about.' Children and parents alike can even end up feeling anxious about feeling anxious!

It's only now that we're beginning to accept that there is an increasing problem of anxiety in children and young people, which is prompting parents and educators to try to tackle it head on. Although awareness of anxiety has increased, far less is known about how to help anxious children. Up to now, the focus has been more on trying to nip anxiety in the bud rather than accepting it as a feeling we all get sometimes. Thankfully this seems to be changing, which reduces the pressure to get rid of it and enables a greater acceptance of it in our lives as something we can learn to manage.

Much like the adults in little Tommy's life, the adults in my life may not have known quite how to help me – but I believe their intentions were good. One of my reasons for writing this book, therefore, is to help parents to recognise anxiety and to acquire the tools they need to help their anxious children by breaking down the walls of miscommunication to navigate a way forward together.

In their shoes[59]

Imagine this. You're travelling along the motorway when your brakes feel as though they might fail. They're working, but something feels off. This has never happened before. You drive the car to the closest mechanic. After a thorough inspection of the car, you're told everything is fine and there's nothing to worry about.

You get back on the motorway and the same thing happens. Your brakes seem to be working, but they don't feel right. You take the car back to the same mechanic, and again, you're told that everything is fine and there's nothing to worry about. You're told this with such certainty that you start to feel a bit silly. Maybe it's not the car or the brakes, maybe it's you.

You're feeling worse now, more confused, and wondering if the problem is actually with you. You get back on the motorway. Your brain keeps reminding you about what happened last time and the time before, and you don't want the same thing to happen again, but it does. You drive to the mechanic and again you're told that everything is fine and there's nothing at all to worry about. You're encouraged to keep driving, which you do, but you avoid the motorway. You're ready to open your loving arms to any explanation that could make sense of your moody brakes. If it's not the car, maybe it's the motorway. Makes sense, right? The easy solution is to avoid it. It would be ridiculous to keep doing the same thing in the same place when it feels all wrong, so that's what you do.

Can you imagine how it would feel when everything inside you is telling you something is wrong, but the person you trust keeps telling you there's nothing to worry about? Now, imagine what would happen if you heard this:

Since you've been avoiding the motorway, the car has been fine. The more you do this, the more certain you are that something about the motorway causes your brakes to feel fragile. This works beautifully: no motorway, no fear of brake failure, no worries … easy, until the day the motorway is unavoidable. You're on the motorway and it happens again. It makes no sense at all and it's terrifying.

This time you find a different mechanic. She looks over the car and says, 'Well it's no wonder you felt as though the

brakes were failing. The car is absolutely fine, it's fabulous
actually, but there's this little thing that happens when the
car is at high speed that causes it to feel the way it does.
It's no problem and it happens a lot with these cars.' As it's
being explained to you, it makes complete sense. Best of
all, it's compelling proof that it's the car that's the problem,
and you're not losing your mind. The mechanic explains
how to stop the car feeling the way it does. She tells you
that this strategy might not work straight away, it can take
a bit of practice, but at least you know what's causing the
trouble, and you can feel safe.

Well, what did you think? What I love most about this metaphor is that it normalises anxiety for children and their
parents, and firmly lays to rest the idea that there's anything
intrinsically wrong with the person experiencing these big
feelings. When I use this metaphor to explain anxiety to
parents, it always seems to hit home, paving the way to a new
understanding.

It paints a picture of how anxiety affects our physical sensations ('your brakes seem to be working, but they don't feel
right'); our thoughts ('you're feeling worse now, more confused,
and wondering if the problem is actually with you'); our
attempts to avoid the problem; ('the easy solution is to avoid
it'); and on the negative cycle this creates ('this works beautifully: no motorway, no fear of brake failure, no worries …
easy, until the day the motorway is unavoidable. You're on the
motorway and it happens again. It makes no sense at all and
it's terrifying').

But consider this: if the child is the driver, the parent is the
first mechanic.

When the first mechanic said everything was fine and there
was nothing to worry about, the child felt lost and confused,
as their body was telling them otherwise. Cue the same

response again, and the child felt there must be something wrong with them. As the feelings got worse, the only solution was to avoid the motorway altogether, which worked up to a point, although it maintained the idea of the faulty brakes.

On the other hand, when the second mechanic took the time to look over the car and explained what was happening, the child felt such relief that they weren't losing their mind and that there might even be some hope that the situation could be improved.

When your child is anxious and something doesn't feel right, *you* are their hope. When they perceive a threat, their body's alarm system is activated, causing a chain reaction of symptoms in their body and in their mind, one of these being to recruit your much-needed support. Because we don't like seeing our kids in pain, parents often feel a huge responsibility to 'fix it', which may prompt them to tell their child that there's nothing to worry about.

The problem is that this chain reaction of mental and physical symptoms is already in motion – and it can't be stopped unless the child is made to feel safe. While parents are desperately trying to make that happen by reassuring their child, what they don't realise is that their child can't process this type of information when they're feeling so unsafe. They need a different type of adult feedback, one that involves addressing what they're feeling right now and riding the wave of anxiety with them without trying to lift them off. Although it's really hard to stay with, the wave won't break them. When we believe it, then they can start to believe it too.

Anxiety made simple

Question: Is anxiety dangerous?

Answer: Anxiety is like a wave. Like any feeling, it will come and then it will go. When the wave comes in, it can feel really scary, as if it's going to drown you. But the reality is that if you ride the wave, by yourself or with someone you love, it won't actually harm you.[60]

Although it feels like one of the most horrible feelings in the world – I know! – it doesn't last long and it goes away after a while, especially if you tell someone how you're feeling, try to ride the wave, take some deep breaths or jump around a few times to let all the tension out. There are lots of calming activities to help you manage anxiety with your child in the Anchoring section and the Appendices.

Experiencing the wave may even make parents and children stronger. Most of all, knowing that it's not your responsibility as a parent to lift them off it – to 'fix' it – might come as a relief. That said, sitting with your child and tuning in to their pain without trying to make the pain go away is far more difficult – but also far more powerful and beneficial to both of you.

Trying to lift your child off their wave of anxiety may even prolong their anxiety, as it could teach them to avoid their feelings or the situations that create them, which limits their experience of life and learning. For any loving parent, the temptation to lift our children out of the way of anxiety can be spectacular. Here's the rub though – avoidance has a powerful way of teaching them that the only way to feel safe is to avoid. This makes sense, but it can shrink their world.

Normalising anxiety:
what your child needs to know

Once you've identified your child as anxious, helping them to understand how anxiety works and the many ways it affects them can help to make it more 'normal' for them – and therefore not as frightening. To know that anxiety is a natural response to a real or perceived threat, and a sign that our strong and healthy brain is doing exactly what it's designed to do to protect us from danger, can help, and to realise they're not the only ones who experience anxiety can be a huge relief.

Psychoeducation: getting the information
you and your child need

The first step of any discussion about anxiety with a clinical psychologist is psychoeducation, which means providing the child (and parents) with accurate information about what it is and how it impacts on them. Explaining that anxiety is a common and normal human experience can reduce a lot of confusion and shame. So too can offering children child-friendly explanations, which can be powerful for them.

Offering your child a simple lesson in what's happening in their brains gives them the power to make choices. Knowledge about the brain can be equally powerful for parents because it means there is a shared language for you to communicate with one another about what's going on. Think of it as your own special language.

All of us get flooded with fear and worry sometimes, which is especially confusing for children, so giving them a vocabulary for their emotional experiences will help them to regulate and manage their emotions.

Anxiety made simple

Question: What's the fight-flight-freeze response?

Answer: Here's a little example, then I'll explain:

> Imagine you're allergic to wasps, and one flies straight into your bedroom through the window. What's the first thing you'd do? If you're feeling up to it, you might find something to kill it with or steer it back out of the window (that's 'fight'). You might run the heck out of the room to shout for help ('flight'). That would be me! Or you might stand totally still ('freeze') until the wasp flies away, because that's what your mum told you is the best thing to do.

The fight-flight-freeze response is automatic – we do it without thinking. It's something we share with animals, and it makes us react immediately to danger without even thinking about it. When faced with a real or imaginary threat, we often feel like our power has been taken away from us. To get our power back, we react in one of these three ways:

- **Fight:** we might get angry, shout, or lash out. This is our way of controlling the threat.
- **Flight:** we might run away or avoid situations. This is our way of controlling what's around us.
- **Freeze:** we might go stiff and feel like our bodies can't move, or that we can't think clearly because our minds have gone blank. This is our way of controlling ourselves.

Many children are relieved to learn that their physical symptoms make sense – that they're neither a sign of them being in serious danger, nor that there is something majorly wrong with them. Naming those feelings with words a child is comfortable using will mean that they can describe what's happening to them when they're anxious. This will help them to feel more grounded and safe. The explanation needs to be short and validating, given that they may not be able to see sense if they're panicked. Take their lead and reflect what you hear and what you see. For example:

'Going into school feels scary for you today. You feel like you've got butterflies in your belly and that you might vomit. This is your fight-flight-freeze response stealing the fuel away from your digestion. That must be really tough for you. Let's try to breathe in some calm together.'

Meerkats, elephants and monkeys

A simple way of explaining anxiety to younger children is using Jane Evans's neuroscience-based 'meerkat brain' model, in which she uses animals to personify parts of the brain:

Little Meerkat, who is good at spotting possible danger and sounding the alarm.

Small Elephant, who is good at working out and remembering the feelings of others.

Mini Monkey, who is great at thinking, planning and calming others down.

In the story, it is Little Meerkat's turn to be on the lookout for any danger to the meerkat gang. All is going well until he falls asleep and wakes up to find that everyone has disappeared, which sends him into one very big panic.

Little Meerkat meets Small Elephant, who is so good at imagining how Little Meerkat is feeling that he joins him in his panic. Next they both meet Mini Monkey, who helps them calm down by taking big breaths in and out together and drinking cool water from the waterhole, after which Little Meerkat is calm enough to explain what happened.

They find the meerkat gang behind a big rock that Little Meerkat had been too panicked to spot earlier. From that day onwards, the three become firm friends, enjoying many adventures together as they have worked out that each has something very special to offer.[61]

Leave the more detailed explanations of anxiety for when your child is calm and best able to take in the information. When you feel calm yourself, ask your child how they have been feeling, and take time to listen and reflect – without trying to make their feelings better. Unpack their worries, and use this as an opportunity to offer a few simple explanations.

Unpacking a worry

Anxiety can feel like a jumbled mess buried deep inside your head, with a presence so gripping that it can be impossible to see the wood for the trees. This is where one of my favourite techniques takes centre stage, which is when the parent attempts to unpack their child's worry in an effort to make sense of this jumbled mess.

In one of my favourite children's books, *The Huge Bag of Worries*,[62] the main character Jenny builds up loads of worries that she carries around with her in a heavy blue bag. The worries are there when she goes to school, when she goes swimming, when she's watching TV, and even when she's in the toilet. She tries ignoring the bag but it doesn't work, and nor does throwing it away or locking it outside her house: 'It was like a horrible shadow she couldn't get rid of,' making her withdraw from her family and toss and turn in her bed all night.

Jenny meets an old lady who asks, 'What on earth is that *huge* bag of worries?' Through her tears, Jenny explains that the bag has followed her for weeks and has become bigger and bigger and just won't go away. The old lady suggests they open the bag to see what's inside. Jenny is reluctant to open it as the worries might jump out at her – and who knows what might happen. The lady says, 'There's nothing a worry hates more than being seen. The secret is to let them out slowly, one by one, and show them to someone else.'

Jenny slowly lets her worries out one by one and is astonished to see how small her bag has become once the old lady has sorted the worries into groups (e.g. those that hate the light of day; those that belong to other people like Mum, Dad or her teacher, etc.). The ending shows a lighter-than-light Jenny and the old lady throwing the bag away. Phew!

This story appeals to me as it's a brilliant metaphor for the hidden worries many children with anxiety carry around with them every minute of every day. What a heavy burden for anyone to carry, especially one that isolates the child from the people from whom they most need comfort and soothing. It's a story about the importance of connection with a close caregiver who remains calm in the face of a child's worries and finds a gentle way to unpack and sort out the jumbled mess of worries in the cold light of day.

Just as in the story, unpacking your child's worries helps both you and your child pinpoint exactly what it is about the particular situation that lies at the root of the worry and enables a deeper exploration into their feelings about it.

Unpacking will also help you see the worry from your child's point of view, which facilitates your feelings of empathy towards them. Your child will feel that you're taking the time to understand their worry and will, in the sharing of their worry, experience relief when hearing the words being spoken out loud.

• •

A case in point: Rose and Lauren

A mother called Rose recounted the story of her nine-year-old daughter, who expressed worries over her parents going away for the weekend while she and her brother stayed with her grandparents. Having overcome serious bouts of anxiety in her earlier years, Lauren was frustrated with herself for feeling so anxious about her parents' trip, and it was made all the worse by not knowing why she was feeling this deep sense of unease.

Mum had noticed that every time the trip was mentioned, Lauren seemed to withdraw and appeared down. Having had a lot of experience in dealing with her daughter's worries before, Mum picked a time when they were both calm and unlikely to be interrupted. Mum sat close to Lauren on the couch and gently brought up what she had noticed:

Mum: Lauren, I noticed that you seem a bit upset every time we talk about me and daddy going away at the weekend. I'm wondering how you feel about it?

Lauren: I'm fine, Mum. Well, no, actually I'm not. I'm so annoyed with myself. I know in my head everything will be fine and I'll be safe. I just hate thinking about your trip and I just don't know how to make it better.

Mum: My poor Laurie. So you feel really worried about us going away for a few nights. You're annoyed with yourself because you know everything will be fine. It sounds like you're struggling with that [Mum holds on to Lauren's hand and takes a few deep breaths to anchor herself and Lauren in the moment and to help her feel understood and connected]. I'm wondering what part of us going away you feel you're most struggling with.

Lauren: I don't know. Maybe all of it. No, not all of it. I'm not worried as much about the weekend as I am about the Friday when we have to say goodbye. Yeah, that's it. It's the Friday I'm dreading.

Mum: So you're more worried about the Friday than the weekend. What do you think it is about the Friday you're dreading?

Lauren: It's the thought of saying goodbye to you at school that really upsets me. All the kids will be around me and I just know no matter how much I try not to I'm going to cry. Then I'll be so embarrassed, and I'll have to spend the whole day in class upset and missing you.

Mum: That's really difficult for you, Lauren. To imagine saying goodbye to me at school and feeling scared that you might cry in front of your friends and be upset for the day [Mum hugs Lauren]. I'm really going to miss you too [Mum waits until Lauren seems calm enough to make a suggestion]. I wonder, would it help at all if we weren't to say goodbye at school and said our goodbyes at home instead?

Lauren: You mean like say goodbye here and then ask Granny to bring me into school?

Mum: Sure, why not? That sounds like a good idea. I could ask Granny and let the school know too. I'm sure it would be OK. Your older brother can make his own decision.

Lauren: Thank you, Mummy! That would be so much better. So that if I get upset, then I'll be able to cry and snuggle into you for a while before going to school and facing everyone.

Mum: You seem so relieved. I'd love to snuggle with you because I know how much I'll miss you and how happy I'll be to see you again on Sunday.

Lauren: Will Granny think my worry is silly, though?

Mum: I very much doubt it. When she was your age, your Auntie Libby got upset every time Granny went for a visit so it's an OK feeling to have and one that Granny is well used to.

Lauren: That's funny thinking of Libby getting upset. Look at her now – she's so ultra brave!

• •

Going back to the SAFE Chain of Resilience which will be elaborated on in Chapter 6: Action, previous to this conversation, Mum took a step back to reflect on whether her own shark music was activated and whether she was calm enough to make her daughter feel safe [**S**elf-care].

In being an emotional anchor, Mum helps Lauren make sense of her anxious feelings by calming her body down and using her body language and voice to make her daughter feel safe [**A**nchoring].

Mum plays the role of emotion detective by unpacking Lauren's worry and reflecting her feelings back in a way in which Lauren felt heard and understood [**F**eeling felt].

Once Mum ensures Lauren feels calm and contained in the moment and meets her needs for safety and love, they come up with a brilliant solution together [**E**mpowerment].

This example may be a milder version of what you encounter, but it gives you a flavour of how naming a scary thing and unpacking it can help a child feel safer. Unpacking also helps to counteract black and white thinking, which is the belief that something or someone can be only good or bad, right or wrong, rather than anything in between or shades of grey, so common in children with anxiety. Using extreme words ('It's all bad') leads children to magnify events through a distorted lens, which ends up making them feel more anxious.

Unpacking a worry helped Lauren to see that there were shades of grey in her perception of the situation, and that the worry wasn't too big when broken down. By talking to her mother, Lauren realised that the thought of her parents' trip wasn't all bad and that only one aspect of it was tricky for her to handle. Her mother stayed with her feelings and wasn't overwhelmed by them. Finding a solution together helped Lauren feel more in control. Processing her feelings in advance of her parents going away helped clear the decks of her mind.

Yes, we have a plan!

Letting children know that anxiety can be managed successfully goes a long way towards reducing both the loneliness and the sense of being overwhelmed that children often feel. Providing your child with an easy explanation of compassion-focused therapy's Three Circles gives you a shared language to talk about anxiety in a more matter-of-fact way, one that acknowledges the beauty of the human brain to consciously move from the Threat circle to the healthier Drive and Soothing circles.

To help you in explaining this to your child, here is a clever analogy introduced to me by consultant clinical psychologist Dr Mary Welford, which compares the Three Circles to mobile phone apps.[63] Mary does a lot of work in the UK to bring CFT into schools, and finds that this analogy works really well with children and teenagers.

Managing emotions: switching our brain 'apps'

Going back to the Three Circles model (see Chapter 1), it can be useful to explain to your child that our brain has three key emotional systems. We can think of these as our brain's 'apps' – the Threat, Drive and Soothing apps. Apps should be familiar to older children as they are so used to the idea of phone apps, how they work, interact – and drain the battery.

It can be helpful to think of our compassionate selves as our operating systems and our emotional regulation systems as applications for our 'smart brains':

Threat

The first circle is the self-protection system, or the Threat app.

Pros
Because our brain is designed to be 'better safe than sorry', the Threat app has a really important role in protecting us from danger and making sure we survive. When we use it, we think and behave in certain ways which can lead to anxiety and other negative feelings (anger, fear, shame) designed to protect us.

Cons
Even though the Threat app is pretty amazing – it will, after all, save our life when there is serious danger – it has two major faults. The first is that it's the biggest battery-drain of all the apps on our phone, particularly when we leave it running in the background. When we

use it too much, our phone ends up totally drained and stops working altogether.

The second problem is that the app just switches on by itself when it thinks there's a threat (when there might not be one) – and when we don't even want it to! So it's a double-edged sword. We can't delete the Threat app from our phones, so we need to find ways to get it to work properly.

The Threat app can get very overactive in people who are anxious because it immediately reacts to threats before any of the other apps get a chance to help it. The Threat app also tricks us into thinking that we should avoid things we're a bit afraid of. The problem is that avoiding things means you never know if it's as bad as you feared (it probably isn't) or if you might surprise yourself by how well you're able to cope (better than you thought, no doubt!).

Drive

The second circle is the achievement system, or the Drive app.

Pros

This is a really enjoyable app to have, because it helps us to play, have fun and use our talents well, and it gives us a buzz for life.

It also reminds each of us of our ability to work hard for the things we want. We all like using the Drive app, because it brings us happiness, fun, excitement and a feeling that we're doing a good job at whatever we're doing.

The Drive app helps us face some of our fears, as long as it joins forces with the magical powers of the Soothing app ...

Cons

Unfortunately, using the Drive app too much can also drain the battery – not as fast as the Threat app, but it does drain it all the same. The secret is not to overuse the Drive app, and to make sure you open the Soothing app at the same time to recharge your battery. This way, you're able to enjoy yourself in school, and do what you like best with your friends and family when you have the energy stored up.

Some kids who feel they have to do things perfectly have their Drive app on all the time, without taking the time to use their Soothing app. When the pressures of school and exams get to be too much, it can be hard to remember to take a break and get some perspective. This helps to turn off the Threat app, so you can use your Drive app when your battery is recharged.

Soothing

Our third and last app is the relaxing Soothing app.

Pros

The Soothing app is there to help us feel safe when we feel anxious. It makes us feel loved, warm, calm and connected with our friends and families. This app helps us to relax, to think positive things and to make good decisions.

What's amazing about the Soothing app is that when we switch it on, rather than drain our battery like the Threat and Drive apps, it magically charges our battery! This is the only app on our phones that the more we use it, the more the battery charges.

The Soothing app is the only one that can stop the Threat app from going crazy trying to fight danger.

The most important job of the Soothing app is to work out whether the danger is real or not, so that it can tell the Threat app to switch off when there's nothing to worry about.

It can also switch off the Drive app if it's been running for too long, because it needs the battery to be fully charged and Drive to be ready when we need to face a fear or do new things.

Cons

Like all the apps, the Soothing app won't work on its own. Most people don't use their Soothing app enough, but if you were somehow able to use nothing but the Soothing system, you wouldn't get anything done! Without a little Drive, we wouldn't get up in the morning; without a little Threat, we wouldn't know when we need to protect ourselves.

Syncing your apps

Just like a smartphone needs loads of apps to perform different functions, our smart brains need all three apps to work well and to keep us healthy.

With smartphones, we switch apps on and off when we need them. With lots of practice, we can do the same with our brain apps. Although the Threat app switches on by itself sometimes, if we use the Soothing app enough, our brains will be calmer and better able to make all the apps work well together.

Ask your child which apps they're using right now, and which ones they use at times when they feel anxious or overwhelmed. Encourage them to practise switching them on and off as they need them, and to think about what might get their

Soothing app working optimally (e.g. more time with friends or family, exercise, sleep, doing something they love).

5
Reflection

Parents are naturally eager to help their children when they're struggling, and parents of anxious children even more so. Having looked at their own anxiety and how that might affect their children's anxiety, readers might now feel primed for action. First, though, it'll pay to think through how anxiety works, how anxious cycles are made, and how anxious ways of thinking are maintained.

As part of this process of reflection, compassion-based therapy asks us to consider how the child's anxiety may have developed. Just as important is understanding what factors are contributing to keeping the anxiety going.

This chapter includes exercises to encourage you and your child to think about anxiety. These try to reshape how you and your child think when you're feeling anxious. Reflection is an active part of anxiety treatment, and is key to managing how we deal with anxiety and its symptoms.

The story of my child's anxiety

Part of my job is to develop a shared understanding with parents and children about how the child's anxiety may have developed and what may be keeping it going. To do this, I create a map of a child's difficulties based on my assessment of the child in their environment. This covers their family, home life, peers, life at school, activities, the wider community and the culture they live in.

I then talk through what I've learned with the child and their parents, whose feedback guides the therapy from there on in.

The simplest way to do this is to use what's called the Five Ps map, which answers the question 'Why is my child having this type of problem, now?' The Five Ps are:

- **Presenting:** What problems does my child seem to be having? How do they affect their daily life?
- **Predisposing:** Why my child? What contributed to the development of the problems? Is it a question of genes; temperament; something that happened when they were younger; the quality of their relationships; their low coping skills; or the culture in which they're being raised?
- **Precipitating:** Why now? What current events might have triggered or fuelled the problem?
- **Perpetuating:** Why is it continuing? What is maintaining the problem? Is my child picking up on fears from other family members? How do others respond when my child is anxious? Has my child been protected from difficult situations and missed opportunities to learn to cope?
- **Protecting:** What strengths can my child draw on? What supports does my child have? Are my child and I motivated to work on reducing their anxiety?

If you'd like to try this for yourself and your child, it may help you to see the big picture of your child's anxiety more clearly, which will help both you and your child to feel empowered going forward. See the Appendix on page 263 for a blank Five Ps map.

As a parent it's difficult for you to be an objective observer of your child's difficulties (neither am I, by the way!), so please only use the above as a tool to reflect on the story of your child's anxiety and what factors may be at play. If your child is really struggling, I would recommend that you seek professional support to help you better understand your child's anxiety.

The four pillars of excess:
creating a less anxious environment

In considering both your own anxiety as a parent and your child's anxiety, you may have started to examine your environment too. This could include your home life and how you spend your time as a family, as well as your work life – your commutes and other commitments. Thinking about all of this might make you anxious, as balancing work and family life these days can be hectic for everyone.

Payne and Ross, in their book *Simplicity Parenting*,[64] describe our modern world as being simply 'too much': there's too much stuff, too much choice, too much speed and too much information. All of this can contribute to us and our children feeling overwhelmed, and lead to a consistent baseline of environmental stresses that build up over time, known as 'cumulative stress reaction'.

On his return from working in refugee camps in South-East Asia, Payne was struck by how children in his private practice in London from what he called 'typical' families presented like the 'wartime kids' he'd got to know in the camps. He was confused to find that despite having what seemed like good lives, the British middle-class children displayed similar levels of nervousness, fight-flight-freeze reactions and over-controlling behaviour as the refugee children.

Whether it was the children in South-East Asia or the children in London, both groups were expressing their anxiety in very physical ways (not sleeping, bedwetting, nightmares, eating issues) and in behavioural ways (clinginess, lashing out, being wary of new situations or changing plans and routines). In coping with their threatening environments, these anxious children were trying to regain control in any way they could, by adopting little rituals around everyday tasks, by being excessively rigid with the rules of a game or activity, and by being distrustful of new relationships, thereby restricting their opportunities to explore and flourish. Payne found that although the British children were physically safe, mentally they were in fact living in a sort of war zone:

> Privy to their parents' fears, drives, ambitions, and the
> very fast pace of their lives, the children were busy trying
> to construct their own boundaries, their own level of
> safety in behaviours that were not ultimately helpful.[65]

Just as the children in the refugee camps were hyper-vigilant and over-controlling due to the wartime traumas they had experienced, the British children appeared to have developed similar coping strategies to help themselves feel safe in managing repeated stresses in their daily lives.

It's worth pointing out that the level of stress described by Payne's cumulative stress reaction is quite different from the stresses that are part and parcel of children's daily lives; it's not a scraped knee, an argument with a friend or five days off with the flu. The paradoxical gift of pain that we covered earlier applies to these day-to-day stresses, ones that, with you by their side, strengthen children's resilience and appreciation of their own abilities.

On the other hand, a cumulative stress reaction comes from consistent and frequent environmental stresses, and is much harder for children to manage. These stresses are what many modern parents call daily life, but such very adult-level stresses can be unwittingly transferred onto children:

A daily life submerged in the same media-rich, multi-tasking, complex, information-overloaded, time-pressured waters as our own. Quite simply: The pace of our daily lives is increasingly misaligned with the pace of childhood.[66]

These environmental stresses collectively compromise a child's ability to be mentally, emotionally and physically resilient. They interfere with a child's emotional baseline of calm, with their sense of security that allows for novelty and change, with their focus and concentration, and ultimately distract from the task of childhood (i.e. an emerging and developing sense of self).

To gain a better understanding of how we can dial down our expectations of ourselves as parents, read on in Chapter 1.

In thinking about how our family lives can be too busy, it's important for parents to take a step back and see how the demands of their own schedule can affect their children. Whether it's too much stuff, too many choices, too much information or too much speed, the sensory overload of these four kinds of 'too much' coming from parents can propel children into becoming more anxious and create an environment in which mental health issues are more likely to flourish.

When children are overwhelmed by what Payne called the four pillars of excess, they lose the precious downtime they need to explore the world, play freely, think and release tension. Some have gone so far as to say that our modern culture of 'too much' is declaring a war on childhood, and that our children's developing brains are struggling to keep up:

Childhood serves a very real purpose. It's not something to 'get through'. It's there to protect and develop young minds so they can grow into healthy and happy adults. When society messes too much with childhood, young brains react. By providing a sense of balance and actively protecting childhood we're giving our children the greatest gift they'll ever receive.[67]

By focusing on simplifying things for themselves and their children, parents can make small, realistic changes to reduce environmental stresses and to reclaim the space and freedom their children need to flourish. Here's how to get started.

Too much stuff

I've a confession to make. I'm a mother who has real difficulty in taking my kids to a toy shop and not caving in to their pressure, even when we're shopping for someone else. Somehow I don't think I'm alone in my plight. As a result, we've a lot of toys in our small house, and it feels like way too much. Interestingly, I've noticed that when we only bring a few well-chosen toys away on holiday, my girls are far more likely to take the time to *really* play with them.

When kids have too much stuff, they become overwhelmed by choice and are more likely to dart from one toy or digital device to another, which overstimulates them and ultimately mimics a fight-flight-freeze response.

Simplicity Parenting encourages parents to keep fewer toys to increase children's attention and their ability to engage more deeply with the ones that they do have. This helps the child to appreciate and focus on what they have, and to spend enough time with their toys to see their full potential for play.

A good starting point is to clear out the clutter and to reduce the number of toys, games, clothes and gadgets in a child's room and in the house, leaving a few all-purpose toys, games and books that you've thoughtfully provided, things that fuel their imagination. This could be a case of moving some stuff out of sight and swapping around what your child has access to on a regular enough basis.

De-cluttering is much easier said than done – you should see under my bed! But if you feel that too much stuff may be contributing to anxiety in your household, then simplifying your child's environment bit by bit, and toy by toy, could help even just a little.

When parents reduce physical clutter in their living space, children's behaviour and mood can improve. The more a child's imagination gets fired up by one little object – say a hula hoop for a circus lion-tamer – the more it engages their creativity and self-directed learning, and the more likely they are to find multiple uses for it.

This encourages the different parts of their developing brain to work in tandem, leading to better emotional health, which is essential as the beginnings of empathy start to take shape. Children are also forced to collaborate better with each other when there are fewer things to play with.

Because our children look to us for guidance, it's also a good idea to become aware of how much stuff *we* have and how much emphasis we place on material belongings. If parents consistently model wanting more stuff, then children will naturally follow suit. What's rare is precious, so teaching them this lesson from an early age is invaluable.

This isn't a new concept, of course – I read Aesop's *The Town Mouse and the Country Mouse* to my girls, and it strikes a similar chord. In it, the town mouse isn't impressed by the country mouse's simple offerings, so he invites him to stay in the mansion he shares with a dangerous-looking dog. Faced with the choice of opulence and danger as an alternative to his simpler life, the country mouse eloquently responds,

'Better beans and bacon in peace than cakes and ale in fear.'[68]

Too many choices

Children's ability to make choices depends not only on their developmental stage, but also on their temperament and state of mind. As with 'too much stuff', kids can become overwhelmed when given too many choices about what they would like or what's happening next. This is particularly true of children who are feeling anxious; they can struggle to make choices because their anxiety directs them towards the 'safest' option, regardless of what they might like or need to do.

An invitation to a birthday party might make a child nervous – what if they don't like the food or don't know all the children? – but they'd probably have a great time if they did go. Sometimes being cautious is the best way to proceed, but equally, sometimes it's not and can interfere with living life to the full.

Anxiety disengages the part of the brain essential for making good decisions – the prefrontal cortex – by reducing its capacity to screen out distractions, which happens because the amygdala becomes overactive. Anxiety also tricks children into believing that there are right and wrong choices, because anxious people tend to practise worst-case-scenario thinking, where consequences are always dire. This can lead to a fear of making the wrong choice: 'What if I choose the wrong thing, and then *this* happens?'

Making decisions

Simplicity Parenting cautions against overwhelming *all* children with choices before they're good and ready. Like most parenting decisions we make, it's about taking a step back and gauging your child's level of development, their state of mind and their ability to make choices. Encouraging choice-making is a way of empowering your child and teaching them to live with the good and bad consequences of each choice, a hugely valuable lesson in life.

It's all about balance, balance and more balance when it comes to offering choices to anxious kids. If you find that your child's anxiety is affecting their decision-making, reduce the number of choices. Left to their own devices, an anxious child may avoid doing things altogether if given too many choices. This reinforces their anxiety as they don't get to face their fears, so finding the right balance is essential.

When there is an important decision to be made, we can all feel a bit pressured. Let your child know that feeling nervous is normal. If they're able to do so, give them the space to make a decision, letting them know that no decision that they come to will be the wrong one. Once the child makes a decision, they can start organising their environment so that what they decided to do is more likely to work out; planning what to bring on a first sleepover, say. And if your child obsesses about things not working out, ask them, 'What's the worst that could happen?' It's usually never as bad as it seems in an anxious child's imagination!

If we encourage children to be guided by what they want rather than what they want to avoid, they're more

> *likely to make a good decision.* Sometimes anxious kids need a gentle push to make a decision, like going to something you know they'll enjoy. Helping them to remember all the times they enjoyed the activity before can be encouraging. Prompting them to imagine how buzzed and proud of themselves they'll feel afterwards can also be a great motivator.

Too much speed

> We live in an age of acceleration. We're cramming our minutes and we're missing our moments. In the rush to the next moment, in the worry about the last moment, we have an awful habit of missing that piece in the middle: our one and precious life.[69]

Speed has become a commodity, and rushing around is now the norm – an adrenaline-fuelled addiction. I once hurried so much to get to an appointment with my own counsellor, that when I finally sat down I thought, 'Ah … now I can relax!' The irony of it – bending over backwards and stressing yourself out in order to take the time to nurture yourself.

Downtime isn't valued in the world we live in, which places more emphasis on speed, money, appearances and success than it does on living in the moment, being true to your values, being good enough and making an effort. The more we focus on achieving pressurised extrinsic goals, the less we focus on nurturing intrinsic goals. This is detrimental to our own and our children's well-being.

Even during those few moments when we do have a chance to unwind, or even when we're waiting for something potentially stressful – such as seeing the doctor or getting our car serviced – many of us, me included, turn towards our devices to check emails and notifications or to see what our virtual friends are up to. By looking down all the time, what are we missing by not looking up?

> We are becoming busier and busier and, as a result, more and more disconnected from the things we need, such as social connection. The growing dependence on social media and internet-based services can lead to disconnection from ourselves and other people.[70]

Disconnecting from ourselves and others is something we as parents should be mindful of, because kids do what they see rather than what they're told. If they see their parents run ragged chasing their tails the whole time, unable to relax in the moment, then they'll think that constant threat-based drive is the norm – and they'll most likely follow suit.

Too many commitments

Not only are parents trying to juggle their own many roles, they often create the same kinds of busy schedules for their children. Because we want to do what we think is best for our kids, we feel pressure to enrol them in countless activities so as not to deprive them or miss an opportunity to nurture potential talent, be it in sport, the arts or any number of extra-curricular activities. We also schedule supervised playdates with military precision; these can be really enjoyable for children, although they can sometimes deny them the opportunity of crucial adult-free play.

And then when kids *do* get downtime, they may well spend it in front of a screen, rather than rejuvenating their Soothing systems. It's generally much better for kids to spend time engaged in free play, unsupervised by adults, which is vital to their healthy emotional, social and intellectual development.

In the tapestry of childhood, it's not computer games and expensive presents your child will most remember, but the repeated threads and rituals individual to your family,[71] like the family dinners, nature walks, card games and bedtime stories.

If you can, take time aside every day to do something which grounds you as a family. These few minutes will reward you all richly.

Too much information

More than ever before, today's children must contend with overexposure to a continuous stream of bad-news stories, such as terrorist attacks, natural disasters and the exploits of less-than-savoury world leaders. They see the shock, anxiety and sadness this causes their loved ones as they constantly check the news on their devices, and they can't but internalise some of this distress. It's a lot for a developing brain to take in.

All of us, children included, go through life believing the world is a safe enough place, otherwise we'd never set foot outside the front door. The anxiety caused by violent events in the world can shake this core belief that the world is a safe place, one which we all rely on.

While any traumatic event can leave adults feeling helpless, children react particularly strongly to events that make them feel unsafe. Children are very aware of their own vulnerability – that they don't have the autonomy or strength to protect themselves. This can get reinforced with every news cycle, particularly so for anxious children whose sense of safety is very easily eroded. Parents are crucial to helping their children understand traumatic events.

For more on how to work through traumatic events with your children, flip ahead to the Appendices, page 243.

Even closer to home than the news on television or social media, there are many adult conversations that children don't need to hear for similar reasons. From worries about money, to parental rows, to their teacher's weaknesses, to stress at work – this is all too much information for a child.

When we discuss adult issues with kids, they come to believe that they're our equals, which can feel overwhelming for them if they aren't developmentally ready. We're their parents, not their friends, so we need to be choosy about what we say and how we say it. Read on to gauge how you might do this by considering the four key questions in the box on the next page.

Too little information

Though there certainly is a danger in children being exposed to too much information, I've also seen the significant impact of children being exposed to too little information.

Almost every child that I meet in my clinic lacks information about something important in their lives. This usually happens for one of two reasons. The first is the parent wanting to protect their child from information that they believe will be too upsetting. The second is that the parent might be at a loss as to how to explain something in a child-friendly way. In both cases, the parents have good intentions.

The problem occurs when children who are not made privy to important information imagine the worst-case scenario. This happens because children naturally have vivid imaginations and have an equally natural tendency to make themselves the centre of everything. It's developmentally normal for children to focus on themselves first – but the downside is that they can blame themselves for situations that have nothing to do with them.

When I was running a group for separated parents, we asked parents to speak to their children about what they understood about the separation. One mother came in the following week and recounted her conversation with her seven-year-old son, who had become upset and said, 'I thought you and Daddy breaking up was all my fault because I'd done a bold thing the day before.' Incredible, isn't it, what kids might believe unless you broach things with them?

If we don't give children an explanation they can understand, they'll come up with their own. Protecting children from conversations parents may not feel comfortable with may actually contribute to kids feeling less safe as they are denied information which is important to their understanding.

This lovely mother wept that her son had believed he was to blame for this for two years, but was relieved that she had finally taken the plunge and managed to explain the separation in a way that he could understand, without his being pressured to take sides.

Too little information? Too much information? The proper degree of separation between the adult world and a child's world is a delicate thing to achieve. Sharing information with your child in a way that acknowledges their feelings and is appropriate to their stage of development is very important, but precisely how much to tell them can be hard to gauge.

Before we say anything about a tricky subject to kids, it can be useful to ask yourself four key questions:

- Is it kind?
- Is it necessary?
- Is it true?
- Will it help my child feel safe?[72]

Unless you can answer yes to all four questions, it may be best to hold back and think before you share. This way you can give your child the information they need to understand their world, but spare them the worries they just don't need to carry. Don't worry if your child asks you a question to which you don't have an immediate answer. You are human too, and it's OK to respond, 'That's an interesting question. I want to think about it before I answer. I'll get back to you when I'm ready.' *And make sure you do get back to them!*

Thinking about anxiety as a cycle

Having considered the whys and hows of anxiety, and worked through some environmental factors that might maintain anxiety, it can help to think about anxiety as a cycle.

Question: What exactly does anxiety consist of?

Answer: To understand anxiety, it's good to know that it's made up of three parts:

- **Thoughts** are what we say to ourselves.
- **Feelings** are how our body reacts.
- **Behaviours** are what we do.

Because our thoughts, physical feelings and behaviours are all related, it's helpful to draw them as a triangle with arrows:

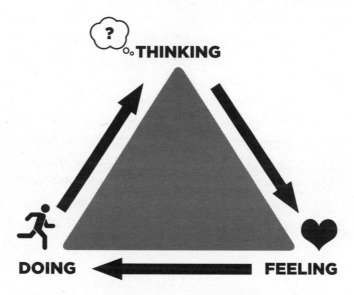

The three parts of anxiety

How we think affects how we feel; how we feel affects what we do; what we do affects how we think. This is a cycle, going around and around again.

The cycle begins with a situation, which leads to a thought, then a feeling, then an action, which then leads back to a thought, and so on.

Breaking a negative cycle is what cognitive behavioural therapy (CBT) is all about. Best used for children over eight, CBT is a talking therapy which focuses on how a person's thoughts affect their feelings and behaviours. By trying to change what we think and what we do to be more positive or realistic, we can shrink our anxious feelings. See exercise on page 216.

A case in point: Ella

There is a child called Ella who has a fear of dogs, stemming from an incident when she once came across a growling dog which frightened her. So every time she sees a dog she thinks it's going to bite her. Having this thought makes her body get ready to fight, run away or freeze. Feeling her heart rate go up and her belly tighten makes seeing the dog even scarier for Ella. As a result, her behaviour changes. She stays away from the park near her house in case she meets a dog, which is sad because she doesn't get to play with her friends there any more. Ella will continue to be afraid of dogs as long as she avoids them:

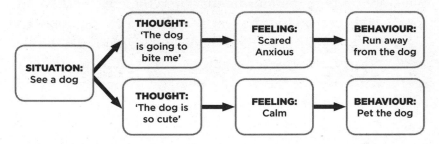

Fear of dogs

Let's come up with a different cycle for the same situation. There is a child called Ella who had once been afraid of dogs but has since met dogs who are friendly and harmless (behaviour). When she meets a little dog, instead of thinking, 'This dog is going to bite me,' she now thinks, 'This dog is so cute' (thought). Having this thought makes her calm and happy (feeling). Ella reaches out to pet the dog (behaviour). Every time she pets a dog, her fear of dogs lessens. She is still a bit afraid of bigger dogs, so that will take a bit more practice.

What changed Ella's thinking about dogs was that her parents encouraged her to face her fear in a very gradual way. They used what is called a 'fear ladder', starting with what she was least afraid of (looking at photos of dogs) and then slowly moving up to what she was most afraid of (standing near a dog at the park). See Appendices for steps on how to make your own fear ladder.

This took a while and wasn't easy, but with plenty of help from her family and friends, Ella realised that the dogs she met were not as scary as she once thought. Once her thoughts changed, her body got the signal to feel more relaxed, and now she's even able to pet a dog!

....

'Nothing is good or bad, but thinking makes it so'

Shakespeare here reminds us that everything we hear, smell, touch, taste and feel in the world is filtered by our thoughts about it. If we see the world as being a dangerous place, then we'll end up feeling scared and avoiding what we think is scary. When we see the world through anxious eyes, lots of things look and feel scary.

If you're stuck in a blizzard, it would be hard to see anything because of all the snow, wouldn't it? If you think of your mind as a snow globe and your scary thoughts as snowflakes, then I wonder what would happen if you shake the snow globe really hard?

All your thoughts would move around, wouldn't they? This is what we call blizzard thinking, and is exactly what happens when we feel anxious. We become blinded by our thoughts and end up 'living in the feeling of our thinking'.[73]

But the great thing is that with lots of practice we can learn to think again. We can also learn to let the snow-flakes gradually settle, and to wake up to the idea that we are not our thoughts and feelings and that we have a choice in how we perceive a situation and respond. Next time your child communicates their worries to you, you could say, 'You've got some really scary blizzard thinking going on right now. That must be really tough. How can we let these thoughts settle before reacting?'

Redirecting anxious thoughts

A good way to help to improve a negative cycle of anxiety is to redirect your negative thoughts. This activity helps parents and children alike to pause and reflect on the kind of thinking which may be feeding their anxiety.[74]

Question: What are *red* and *green* thoughts?

Answer: An easy way to remember the difference between helpful and unhelpful thoughts is to imagine traffic lights:

- **Red means Stop!** This is because the thought is unhelpful, negative and worrying. A red thought makes us think the worst about a situation, which can be upsetting. Examples of red thoughts are: 'Nobody likes me'; 'I'm no good at this'; 'I'll never feel OK again'; 'I won't tell anyone how I feel because no one will care.'
- **Green means Go!** This is because the thought is helpful, positive and powerful. A green thought can help us to feel strong inside, and brave and calm. Examples of green thoughts are: 'I'm a great friend'; 'I'm safe'; 'I can totally do this'; 'My parents/teacher can help me'; 'Everyone has their own special talents.'

When faced with a difficult situation like being asked to speak up in class, a first reaction might be to have an unhelpful red thought like, 'Oh no, the kids are going to laugh at me.' This ends up making us feel bad and a bit bossed around by our own thoughts, like we can't do anything about how things will turn out.

Instead, in the same situation, it's possible with practice to choose a more helpful green thought like, 'I'll make sure to breathe and read slowly. The last time I read, nobody laughed.' This makes us feel better and more in control of the situation.

Green thoughts are worth paying attention to because they enable us to do things we're a little afraid of and help build resilience.

From now on, when you or your child have a red thought in response to a situation, once you have acknowledged the red thought and the feeling behind it, have a go at finding an alternative green thought for it. Maybe try this yourself first, then try it out with your child when you are both calm: 'So you feel sad because "No one said hi to me today". That's hard for you, pet. [Parent gives child a hug.] Remember we talked about red and green thoughts? I wonder, could we come up with a green thought for what happened? How about "Today, it seemed like my friend didn't say hi to me, but maybe she didn't see me or had something else on her mind. I put my head down after that and didn't see if anyone else said hi. People usually say hi and want to play with me so I will try again tomorrow".'

 To see this in action, flip ahead to Learning to think green thoughts on page 265.

6
Action

Getting started: your important role

As we've seen, anxiety is the result of all the things which cause us stress minus our beliefs about our ability to cope. When a child feels under threat, they'll constantly look to their parent to check how big the threat really is, as they're not in the best place to evaluate it themselves. Parents are the most important agents for change in helping their children overcome difficulties with anxiety.[75]

Because parents play a huge role in helping their children to regulate their emotions, it follows that during their most anxious moments children look to their parents for help in evaluating the threat. If the parent responds in an anxious way, the child will most certainly remain immobilised. If the parent tunes in and exudes calm, then the child is more likely to get back to a more regulated state.

Part of helping a child back to safety is tuning in to them using your soothing words and actions, and helping them to understand what may be happening for them. During an anxious moment, what your tuning in and reflection does is to communicate to them that you 'get' what they're feeling, that what they're feeling makes sense, and that they're safe. This is only possible if you try to remain calm yourself and respond with compassion.

> Anxiety is contagious, but so is calm, especially your soothing calm.

As you'll see, following the steps of the SAFE compassionate approach restores your child's belief in their ability to cope, thereby creating a more empowered way forward.

Building the SAFE Chain of Resilience

As I was writing this book, this simple formula kept going around my head on repeat:

> Anxiety + Compassion = Resilience

The fact that anxiety came to visit your child's life was certainly not something that you asked for. However, responding to your child with compassion in your heart and in your mind is something that you *can* work on. I've no doubt that there are many ways in which you're already helping your child to manage; it's about figuring out what's working well and what could be improved on.

When anxiety rears its scary head, compassion helps to calm a child in the moment, and over time, helps to build their expectation that communicating their need to you will be met with your support. Meeting a child's anxiety with compassion builds their resilience as it strengthens the pathways in their brains connecting help-seeking with soothing from loved ones. This in turn helps them to self-soothe in the face of threat as they grow older. Learning to approach your child's anxiety with little gems of compassion, including kindness, feeling your common humanity, and mindfulness as you ride the wave can act as a useful framework for exploring anxiety, be it your child's or your own big feelings. Focusing on nourishing your own and your child's Soothing circles reduces the power of the Threat circle so you can approach life with wonderment rather than fear. In this way, compassion is truly at the heart of empowerment, learning and inner strength.

Compassionate parenting in action

Compassion facilitates connectedness and builds social relationships through caring behaviour;[76] is essential to the development of secure child–parent attachment relationships; and has been found to lower stress, anxiety and low mood, while improving self-worth and resilience.[77] Pretty powerful stuff!

At the heart of compassionate parenting is the connection between the parent and child, a connection that is focused on the value of emotions.

> If we can start to see that our emotions are part of the human experience, alerting us to potential difficulties in our lives, then we can start to move towards them and work effectively with them. There is an idea that emotions are a sign of weakness, something to be ignored and avoided. As a result of these messages, people don't value their emotions; they don't see their emotions as the friends that they are, trying to alert them to problems in their lives and unmet needs.[78]

Our emotions have a heck of a lot to teach us – if only we'll let them. A compassionate approach requires us to slow right down and try to see what lies behind our child's feelings and behaviour. I call this the 'secret message'. This can be difficult when parents are struggling with their own emotions, because their feelings can get in the way of understanding the message behind their child's feelings.

At times, many of us (me included) walk around think-ing we're not doing such a good job of this parenting business – especially when we're struggling to help our child. But the irony is that berating ourselves actually gets in the way of understanding what our child needs.

Treating ourselves with compassion and under-standing enables us to do the same for our children. In this way, we help them to feel safe, understood and empowered. Learning to be kind to ourselves carries huge benefits for parents and children alike.

A kind heart can:

- Explore any of your own discomfort provoked by your child's anxiety, and work on feeding your Soothing circle with **S**elf-care.
- Realise your crucial role in **A**nchoring your child, while encouraging their gradual exposure to the things they fear.
- Connect to your child's kind heart to unpack the secret message behind their anxiety, helping them feel accepted and understood – **F**eeling felt.
- Build your child–parent relationship from which a range of empowering and problem-solving strategies can emerge – **E**mpowerment.

There are many benefits of compassion and compassion-focused therapy (CFT) for parents.

I discovered CFT helping with the management of my depression and my approach to parenting. It made so much sense and I could see how I had been sustained by Drive and Threat without ever really stopping to be with myself or to nurture my Soothing. As a parent of teenagers I wish I'd discovered it earlier. I think key changes are recognising that it's OK to be nervous and worried about how you're doing as a parent, that it's a common feeling and sometimes we all find it overwhelming. For my children I hope that I'm helping them to be more engaged with and understand their emotions, increasing their openness to talk about how they feel so they don't have to go through the really tough times that I did.[79]

All parents struggle – which is one of the things that gives us our common humanity. Knowing this can enable us to be more aware of our feelings and accepting of our vulnerabilities (self-kindness), which in turn helps us to welcome our children's feelings (mindfulness), which makes them more able to share these feelings openly with their parents.

 If you're having a hard time being kind to yourself, try the *Love in, love out* meditation for parents in the Appendices, page 252.

Compassion asks us to be gentler to ourselves, and to gently encourage our harsh inner critic to become a softer, more understanding voice. Compassionate parenting is about bringing kindness into our relationship with ourselves rather than self-criticism, because this doesn't do anyone any good. By turning down our critical voice it helps to know that we're all in the same boat with our struggles and that we can use our vulnerabilities to create a better connection with our children in a more wholehearted way, which sees vulnerability as lying at the centre of the family story:

> [Vulnerability] defines our moments of greatest joy, fear, sorrow, shame, disappointment, love, belonging, gratitude, creativity, and everyday wonder. Whether we're holding our children or standing beside them or talking through their locked door, vulnerability is what shapes who we are and who our children are.[80]

If we refuse to be vulnerable during moments of struggle and self-doubt, rather than *being* with ourselves through the peaks and valleys of life, we'll struggle to teach our children to acknowledge their own vulnerabilities.

Parents' feelings about themselves are vital to raising children who live and love with their whole hearts. If we want our children to love and accept who they are, then we must love and accept who we are *including* our imperfections:

> We can't use fear, shame, blame, and judgment in our own lives if we want to raise courageous children. Compassion and connection – the very things that give purpose and meaning to our lives – can only be learned if they are experienced. And our families are our first opportunities to experience these things.[81]

Our own vulnerabilities and those of our children – far from being something to hide – provide us with precious moments to explore our colourful emotions with our children, to develop love and compassion, and to teach them resilience from a place of being 'good enough' rather than equating vulnerability with weakness.

Naturally, you would not wish for your child to struggle with anxiety – or anything else, for that matter. But struggles are normal and struggles are *necessary*. Your child's struggle happens to be anxiety. Whilst that's really difficult for them and for you, you're now armed with the knowledge that there *is* a way to convert anxiety into emotional resilience: with your compassionate response to their struggles.

Welcoming anxiety

I would even go so far as to say that now anxiety is present, perhaps you could open the door and welcome it in. Given how tough your child has had it, and that you're probably feeling lost at sea with it, I know this is a long shot. But reframing anxiety's presence in your lives could well be a crucial 'survive-and-thrive'[82] moment, where really difficult moments are seen as opportunities to help children manage them.

- The key to an emotionally healthy life is resilience, which means learning to cope with manageable threats and to rebound in the face of difficulties.
- The single most important factor in developing resilience in children is at least one stable, committed and trusting relationship with a close adult. Children need someone to turn to in challenging times because a child's capacity for self-soothing is born out of repeated instances of being soothed by their parent.
- A parent's compassionate response to their child during their anxious moments has the power to deactivate their Threat system and activate their Soothing system. The calmer and

safer a child feels, the more access they'll have to their Soothing system, which over time enables them to better evaluate and manage future threats.

- A child–parent relationship characterised by compassionate support and emotional regulation promotes resilience and is a necessary part of good mental health. The quality of the child–parent attachment bond provides children with a psychological immune system for dealing with stressful situations in the future and promotes emotional well-being.

Regulate – relate – reason

It's important to respond to an anxious child in a way that complements how their brain takes in information. It's equally important to remember that children simply don't have access to the reasoning part of their brain when they're anxious, because their mind and body are screaming at them that there's a threat. When a child perceives a real or imagined threat and they get into fight-flight-freeze mode, stress chemicals shut down the reasoning part of the brain to protect it and to focus the body's energy on reacting quickly. After all, who needs to think when they're being chased by a lion! This is why reasoning with a child mid-anxiety attack doesn't often work and indeed can often make them even more anxious.

Never in the history of calming down has anyone ever calmed down by being told to calm down.

Telling an anxious child to calm down or reassuring them that everything will be OK goes against what their brains and bodies are telling them. The same is true for us. Showing impatience or frustration can also make the situation worse, as your child then no longer feels safe confiding in you about their anxiety, leaving them feeling alone and afraid that you're overwhelmed too.

Containment is a parent supporting their child to feel safe with their emotions. In order for parents to be able to contain their children's anxious feelings, parents need to feel contained themselves, which is related to how they care for themselves.

A parent's ability to contain their child's anxiety restores the child's ability to think. When a child is mid-anxiety, their ability to think goes offline, so it's the parent's responsibility to get it back on stream. If a parent is struggling with big feelings of their own, then this is likely to impact on their ability to contain and nurture their child's sense of safety.

Researchers in the area of trauma have given us great insight into how to respond to children who feel threatened or unsafe: they need safety and soothing *before* reasoning and problem-solving. The Three Rs[83] describe this sequence:

Am I safe?

Regulate: We must help the child to regulate and calm their fight-flight-freeze responses, and offer soothing comfort.

Am I loved?

Relate: We must connect with the child through a sensitive relationship with them by empathising and validating their feelings so they feel seen, heard and understood.

What can I learn from this?

Reason: Once a child is calm and connected, we can support the child to reflect, learn, remember, articulate, problem-solve and become more self-assured.

SAFE Chain of Resilience

In times of stress, you play a crucial role in containing your child's anxiety, finding the tricky balance between helping them to feel safe and empowering them to test their fears and solve problems. To find this balance, I have developed the four steps of the SAFE Chain of Resilience to support you in navigating your child's anxiety.

The idea behind the SAFE Chain of Resilience came to me as I was thinking about how the chain that connects the anchor to the ship could serve as a metaphor for the parent being a child's emotional anchor. Connected by the chain, the boat can only drift so far in any direction around its centre.

This emotional anchor is provided through a relationship with a sensitive parent who meets the child's needs and to whom the child can turn as a safe haven when upset or anxious or as a secure base from which to face new challenges. Sensitive, compassionate parenting calms the child's anxiety over time and builds resilience.

In developing an approach based on how a child's brain takes in information, I took inspiration from the Three Rs, but focused first on self-care. This provides a chance to introduce another R – reflection – which parents need to do in considering how they look after themselves and regulate their own emotions. This step is absolutely crucial, which is why it comes first.

Self-care: How you look after yourself as a parent and regulate your emotions. **Reflect** on this.

Child: Is my parent contained enough to contain my anxiety?
Parent: I'm emotionally available for you.

Anchoring: How you can help your child feel safe and secure, knowing that you're there for them. Help your child to **regulate** their emotions.

Child: Am I safe?
Parent: You are safe.

Feeling felt: Help your child feel connected and understood by **relating** to them.

Child: Am I loved?
Parent: I'm here with you.

Empowerment: Give your child the tools to manage their anxiety by **reasoning** through it with them.

Child: What can I learn from this?
Parent: We can find a solution together.

To summarise, tuning in to your own needs as a parent facilitates you being able to anchor your child to safety and connect with them, which empowers them to cope with manageable threats. It is all about responding to a situation with love for them and with love for you.

Self-care

I still remember wheeling my trolley around the ward, looking in at my precious baby girl, tears of joy and sadness streaming down my face. What was wrong with me? Why couldn't I hold it together? The most amazing thing had just happened to me, the very thing I had been hoping for all of my life – to become a mother – and I just felt so overwhelmed by my emotions and petrified of the massive responsibility that lay ahead.

I quickly came to realise the enormity of becoming a parent in the hours and weeks after having my first child. The most poignant aspect was the huge sense of responsibility for this little baby looking up at me. Oh boy, how was I going to meet her needs – not just now but forever more? How would I cope with so little sleep? Would my life ever return to normal again? Was I actually going to be able to do this at all when I felt so fragile myself?

Parenting is a complete rollercoaster ride from conception to forever. Nothing can compare to the enormity of a person's transition to parenthood. Parenting an anxious child is even more challenging. Remember: you're doing a really tough job in containing your children's big emotions while often feeling overwhelmed yourself.

Most children's needs reduce with age from those first nerve-wracking weeks, or at least develop to the point where a parent is not needed quite as much. But when you have a child with anxiety, it's like the invisible cord between you grips even tighter whenever they encounter a novel or feared situation. Totally natural then for your stores of strength and patience to be depleted.

To add insult to injury, in this information age we live in, we are bombarded by messages about how to parent our children, which can feel overwhelming and are not always scientifically informed. Although 'it takes a village to raise a child', the village is gradually getting smaller, sadly leaving parents with less social support than ever before during a time of real vulnerability.

Parenthood: the great leveller

In describing a person's transition to parenthood, my colleague once described it as the great leveller, which really resonated with me. It doesn't matter who you are or where you live, making that transition into the unknown of having children is a very big deal.

> No matter who you are in your day-to-day life, once you or your partner becomes pregnant, there is no PhD or CEO position that can get you out of what is ahead. Parenting is the great leveller; once you have a child you are a parent, and we all have much in common in that role regardless of all the other roles we have in life. Your child will always see you as Mum or Dad, [irrespective] of how people outside your four walls see you. It's the primary connection.[84]

Without good social support and evidence-based information about what children need, the transition to having children can make new parents even more vulnerable. What makes it harder still is that society's expectations are higher than ever before, as are the expectations we place on ourselves to be the perfect parent. Too much advice and pressure, and too little social support, has been contributing to parental anxiety, which can leave us in the state of mind so eloquently (!) described here:

> Caught somewhere between OMG and WTF, we feel stuck without any kind of reference point we can trust.[85]

If this chimes at all with how you may be feeling right now, you're not alone. There are many parents struggling out there, watching their children struggle, having tried so many ways to help them, who end up feeling lost and powerless – and that is very scary for a parent, feeling not good enough. I hear echoes of these feelings of inadequacy in my clinic time and time again, and I feel it myself at home – that I could be doing a better job of it, that I'm not maternal enough, the list goes on ...

But you know what? My realisation that I also have needs that deserve to be recognised so that I can give my best to my children has been transformative.

Why is parental self-care so important?

Parenting takes up a *lot* of energy and a *lot* of patience. Parents feel pressured to give so much of themselves to their children that they can often forget to look after their own needs or feel guilty for even considering them. But this is counter-productive, and I'll tell you why.

When a parent neglects to look after themselves they're putting undue stress on their minds and their bodies. This stress can lead to emotional effects such as being irritable, exhausted or sad, but it can also lead to physical effects like a weaker immune system and high blood pressure. I'm sure you've noticed when you're not taking care of yourself that you're more likely to have a short fuse and feel overwhelmed by your children's needs.

Anxiety made simple: self-care

To be a calm, loving and empathetic parent, you need to take good care of yourself. You are your best resource, so it's imperative that you look after yourself. You can't give to your child if you don't have the capacity to give, nor can you contain their big emotions if you feel emotionally overwhelmed or lack crucial support yourself.

Parental self-care is about achieving balance and filling your cup so you have something to give in each of the many roles you play in your life, be it mother, father, spouse, partner, child, friend, worker or carer. Self-care means recognising your feelings and taking the time you need to restore physical, mental, emotional, spiritual and social balance.

Having this balance will enable you to take a step back from your child's anxiety to decide on the best way forward. Ultimately, it will help you to build your confidence as a parent. If you're feeling overwhelmed or drained, you'll be less able to contain your child during a moment of distress and to practise the much-needed pause of *Love in, love out* to anchor you and your child to safety.

On the other hand, if you take a proactive approach to nurturing your self-care, you're far more likely to have the physical and emotional reserves to take on the unpredictability of what each parenting day brings.

You may not know this, but your child is your greatest admirer and is constantly on the lookout for how you manage situations. Consider for a moment the following questions:

- 'What happens to my child when I neglect self-care?'
- 'What tone would I like to set in my everyday interactions with my kids? Calm? Nervous?'
- 'What would I like to model to my child about valuing themselves enough to prioritise their own well-being?'
- 'How will my attitude and actions impact on how my child copes with the inevitable ups and downs of life?'

When we as parents neglect self-care, we're teaching our children that it's OK to put everyone else first, that it's OK to disregard our own needs and that it's OK to ignore other important relationships in our lives (e.g. with partners, family and friends). Parenting can then become an even greater challenge than it already is, as we're not getting the energy we need to do the job well, nor are we availing ourselves of the support we need to fill our emotional cup.

For these reasons, engaging in self-care is a really important life skill that is not only vital for you but also for your child. By feeding our Soothing circle, we're showing our children how best to manage stress and be resilient. We are teaching them that adults have self-care needs that are worthy of being met – and children have them too. We can then encourage them to find ways of meeting those needs and to ask for help in doing it.

One of the aims of a group I ran for parents of anxious kids was to encourage them to engage in a bit of self-care between sessions. This might include going for a walk, having a chat with a friend or attending a yoga class. I could feel some of their stares hardening when the group heard me focusing on nurturing self-care activities rather than offering answers to their various dilemmas. It was totally understandable frustration on their part, but there was a method to my madness!

Engaging in self-care was really hard for many in the group, because they felt so depleted from managing their anxious children's worries.

Unfortunately, a vicious cycle had begun to form for a number of them, looking something like this:

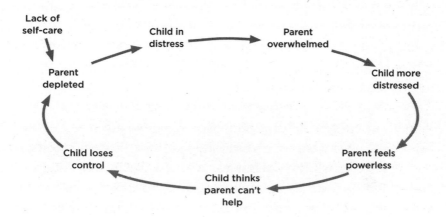

The notion of self-care usually takes a back seat during times of parenting stress, which is understandable; your first instinct is to want to help your distressed child, rather than look at filling your own cup. Focusing on yourself may even seem counter-intuitive.

But can you see how filling your own cup actually helps you to help your child? It enables you to calm yourself, to reflect on your feelings, to come to see what your child requires and to decide how to respond in a way that meets both your needs.

The greatest lesson I have learned since becoming a parent myself and from working really closely with parents is that self-care cannot be ignored and needs to take pride of place in every family home. Looking after your needs as a parent is not selfish – it's fundamental to us all:

Taking care of yourself doesn't mean me first, it means me too.

L. R. Knost

● ●

A case in point: Anita and Luke

Anita, the mother of an anxious child called Luke, bravely shared her feelings with me. 'I don't even like myself,' she said. 'I'm not a good enough mum. Parenting just doesn't come as naturally to me as it does to others. I'm scared Luke is picking up on all my insecurities and it's all my fault.'

Hearing these words made me feel so sad for Anita, as I had learned about her difficult early home life, where many of her emotional needs were not consistently met, which impacted on how she viewed herself throughout her life. She was highly critical of herself, feeling quite alone in her struggles and sure that, no matter what she did, Luke would end up insecure like her. She blamed herself for her son's anxiety and for not knowing how to help him.

Focusing my attention solely on Luke would not have been as fruitful without first exploring Anita's history with her and trying to build up her self-compassion. When children enter therapy, they need the containment of at least one stable parent or loved one to be their support through the journey. Luke was better able to delve deeper when he felt free to lay aside his worries about his mother. I felt that Luke would most benefit from having his mother reflect on her own childhood story and how this impacted on her parenting, before seeing Luke for sessions on his own. In this way, I became Anita's 'container' to free up her space to contain Luke's emotions.

As I'd done with Jonathan on the *Stressed* documentary, I asked Anita to draw her three circles. She drew the Threat and Drive circles really big. When asked about her Soothing circle, she looked at me bewildered and replied, 'What's that? I don't know what that means.' Sadly, she was unable to identify what she found soothing in her life. 'How do I increase my Soothing circle if I don't feel worthy of love?' she asked. 'How do I help my son to nurture his if I can't do it for myself?'

In Anita's case, we discovered that her need to keep busy all the time (Drive) came from a really painful part of her childhood (Threat), during which most of her negative emotions were ignored or denied, as they lay outside of her parents' comfort zones. It became apparent that Anita had never learned how to soothe herself from either of her parents when she was growing up, so she now struggled to identify her own Soothing circle.

It's worth saying that in no way were we blaming her parents for what had happened; these transgenerational patterns generally make sense – reasons can be given for them – when considered in context.

Just like her mother who rarely took a break, Anita had learned how to repress difficult feelings by making sure that she was always doing something, because the alternative, being idle, would have given her too much time in which to think about past pain. Interestingly, his mum being constantly busy came up during play sessions with Luke. Ultimately, he felt that she didn't have time to listen to his worries and help him to figure them out. Anita agreed that she found it very difficult to sit still with Luke's anxiety: 'I've no idea what to say to him – it all feels like too much.'

Working with Anita in addition to working with Luke might have taken twice as much time, but it yielded more than twice the meaningful results for Luke and his mother. My role was to help Anita to recognise her shark music, to teach her how to support herself and assist Luke through his anxious moments, and to focus on nurturing their relationship. Thankfully, their relationship had become much stronger by the end of my time with them. Although difficulties still came up, I knew they would be better able to manage them together. Given that Anita had difficulty sitting still for long, we agreed that Luke could share his worries with her for ten minutes each day during 'worry time', after which they would leave it until the following day. I helped Anita with breathing techniques so that she could welcome Luke's feelings without becoming overwhelmed by them.

The value of working on yourself

'Each of us is a beautiful mess. We can pretend to be
perfect alone or admit that we're messy together. Messy
together is better.'[86]

I love this quote because it captures the struggles that all
parents face. There is a beauty in being human and knowing
that we're all on this bumpy ride together. When we share our
struggles, we gain a clearer perspective on what we have in
common rather than what divides us, which ultimately helps
us to be kinder to ourselves.

I have met a lot of parents who don't feel good enough about
themselves and beat themselves up for every perceived inadequacy. While they may have already had their struggles
pre-kids, becoming a parent has magnified their feelings
threefold, and they're lost in a sea of negativity and self-blame.
It's heartbreaking that they don't see the beauty that I see and
even more heartbreaking that they don't see the beauty that
their adoring children see.

Each of us comes into our parenting role with a certain
amount of emotional baggage that we might not have processed.
Sometimes it's only when we become parents that our old
scripts from the past re-emerge and we're suddenly faced with
seeing them repeated in our interactions with our children.
Having kids pushes us to take a long hard look at ourselves and
we may not always feel comfortable with what we see.

Before I had kids, I had gone to counselling a good bit to
work through various issues from my past which were still
impacting on me. However, it was only when I became a
parent that I realised there were a few extra skeletons which
had never seen the light of day!

There is no escaping our past no matter how much we try.
Over the course of our lifetime, we build up defences to keep

our childhood pain at bay (e.g. denial, acting out, over-control). Unfortunately they only work for a limited time and can end up falling to pieces when faced with the gruelling challenges of parenting.

Working on yourself is one of the best investments you can make as a parent, not only for you, but for your kids. When I begin to work with parents on deepening their awareness of how their past may have impacted on how they see themselves now, a light bulb goes off. It can be harder for some than others depending on their stories and self-awareness.

> Becoming a parent affords you an incredible opportunity to grow as an individual, knowing that this self-growth will benefit you, your child and your relationship.

All parenting begins with you. How you relate to yourself has a huge bearing on how you relate to others, including your child, and on how they view themselves. You are a mirror to their feelings about themselves. Now that we know that children model their behaviour on their parents, can we really encourage children to love themselves if we don't love ourselves in turn? This is not about high-fiving ourselves in the mirror every second of the day; it's about nurturing a deep acceptance of ourselves, including our imperfections.

Considering this important link, I wonder if you took a moment to look into the mirror to really see yourself in your entirety. What do you see?

- Do you often have a sense of your lovability as a person and a belief that you're good enough just as you are?

- Or do you find yourself operating from a place of fear and insecurity?
- Do you accept mistakes as part of your parenting journey from which to learn?
- Or do you perceive mistakes as just another way in which you are failing as a parent?

Your answers are reflected in how you look after yourself on a daily basis and whether you feel deserving of self-care. If this is difficult for you, this may stem from your early experiences of being cared for, which may well be worth exploring a bit further.

If you haven't already addressed any of your own anxieties or pain from the past, now is a good time to start, in whatever small way you can. If you find that a certain issue keeps coming up time and time again, or that you have a strong reaction to your child expressing their needs, then it may be beneficial to speak to a professional psychotherapist or psychologist who can help you to explore those issues.

When picking someone to help you and your child, make sure they're accredited in their field and that they have suffi-cient experience. If you don't click with the first therapist you meet, try another. It's really important to find someone that you connect with and in whose company you feel comfortable. Going to see a therapist may not be for everyone. However, seeking support, whether through a professional or through more informal channels, like talking to friends or family, is known to have significant benefits in helping parents fill up their emotional cup – so do try to find the best support you can.

Valuing yourself enough to look after your own well-being can be really challenging for many parents for many different reasons, as discussed already. But here's the newsflash: *it's OK to do things for yourself!*

As a parent of an anxious child, it's of paramount importance that you look after yourself both for your own well-being and for that of your child. And yet I know how hard it is to prioritise self-care among all the competing priorities you face, not least the considerable needs of your child.

I remember the day a worried couple came into my clinic all ready to learn strategies to help their anxious child, and just before leaving were surprised to learn that one of my recommendations was: 'Given that you haven't been out together in the last eight years, I'm prescribing that you go out – just the two of you – for a few hours between now and the next session.'

The reason I did this was that I could sense that their focus was so much on their anxious child that they had somehow lost a bit of a connection as a couple, which was impacting on their ability to agree on a joint approach in response to their child. Thankfully, they came back for the next session a little bit more relaxed and ready to tackle how to best help their child together.

This is what SAFE is all about – it's about laying the firm foundations for you as a parent so you're better able to meet your child's need for containment, connection and calm. Read on to learn more about how you can do that using the lotus of self-care I have specially designed with you in mind.

Self-care

Lotus of self-care

I have come to believe that caring for myself is not
self-indulgent. Caring for myself is an act of survival.

Audre Lorde

We cannot care for our children unless we get the time to
recharge our batteries. This is the first action that we need to
take. Every one of us has a different recharge mechanism – it's
simply a matter of finding what works for you and really prioritising the time to do it on a regular basis. By taking care of
yourself, you'll be happier in yourself, have more to give, and
everyone in your family will benefit.

Parental self-care isn't a one-time chore that you need to
tick off so you can get on with the next item on your long list.
It's the *intentional* care of your physical, psychological,
emotional, spiritual and social well-being through repetition
of everyday practices. Together these elements combine to
nurture you as a human being and as a parent, and facilitate
you functioning at your optimum.

In thinking about self-care, I am hugely drawn to the
Buddhist mantra 'Hail to the Jewel in the Lotus' found on a
ring my husband acquired on one of his great Indian adventures. The lotus is a hugely powerful symbol used in many
Eastern traditions on account of its unique properties. The
plant grows up from the muddy bottom of a pond, from which
it must push hard and work its way through the muck and
water until it eventually breaks the surface of the pond and
blooms elegantly in the nurturing sunlight, dancing up and
down with the changing current. The lotus is beautiful in
colour and smells divine. Although it grows out of the murky

darkness of the pond, it brings beauty and light, hence the saying, 'No mud, no lotus'.[87]

In the Buddhist tradition, the fruit, the flower and the stalk of the lotus symbolise the passage of time: the past (stalk), the present (flower) and the future (fruit). Equally prized is the jewel in the flower – the seed – which is the potential within all of us, which I consider to be a coming together of wisdom and practice. The wisdom comes from learning from our past vulnerabilities, while the practice is the lotus itself, which is the self-care plan we need to create for ourselves.

Another symbolic characteristic I love about the lotus is that the plant's stalk is easy to bend in two but is very hard to break because of its many strong and sinuous fibres. Chinese poets use this as a metaphor for the close and unbreakable relationship between family members, showing that no matter how far away they are nothing can separate them in their hearts.

This ties in so beautifully with the analogy of the parent being an emotional anchor to their child and the invisible cord that forever exists between them, even through muddy waters.

Similarly, in nurturing yourself to support and contain your anxious child through their muddy waters, it's important to set the intention to refill your cup, to show yourself kindness and compassion, and to actively manage and reduce your daily stresses.

It's about finding the method that works best for you and your child using your inner wisdom, and figuring out what supports you need to help you to achieve this.

And always remember that *it's OK to ask for help*, because getting started often means asking others for practical and emotional support.

Five dimensions of self-care

The reason I chose to represent self-care with the five-petal lotus flower is that there are five dimensions of health: physical, psychological, emotional, spiritual and social. The flower is a meaningful metaphor because its petals joined together make a balanced whole.

Consider for a moment which self-care activities you currently prioritise in each area of your life:

• How do you nourish your body, heart, mind, spirit and social selves on a regular basis?
• What realistic plan can you make to nurture each of these areas of your health?
• Once you can identify at least one plan for each area, what support do you need to make it happen?

If it helps, try to remember a time when you felt invigorated by something you were doing or by people you spent time with, where time stood still as you blissfully engaged in something or with someone that you truly valued.

If you can't think of anything that really floated your boat recently (these memories can sometimes be hard to find when you have kids!), think of something that really resonated with you in your earlier years.

For many, this could be engaging in free play and exploring the wonders of the world through innocent eyes. For others, this could be the soothing and warmth you got from a close family member, teacher or friend when you most needed it.

Whatever your memories, try to take valuable lessons from them about what makes you the unique human being that you are, with your very own soothing 'data bank' of memories that anchor you. This will nurture your Soothing circle with feelings of peaceful well-being, connection and contentment.

Remember, it's our focus on the Soothing circle that helps to calm and balance the Drive and Threat circles, triggering the release of the love hormone oxytocin, which fine-tunes our social instincts and strengthens close relationships.

Nourishing your Soothing circle not only replenishes you as a parent, but it positively impacts on your capacity to reflect on and respond to your child's needs.

Anxiety made simple: give yourself a break

Please don't underestimate the impact of using a kind and gentle tone of voice when relating to yourself. If you don't use warmth in your relationship with yourself, self-care activities become just another chore, something that has to be done as opposed to an act of love.[88]

If it all feels a bit overwhelming, try to start small and welcome tiny self-care habits into your life every day, so that you can give your body, your mind and your soul the little bit of love and attention it so much craves and deserves.

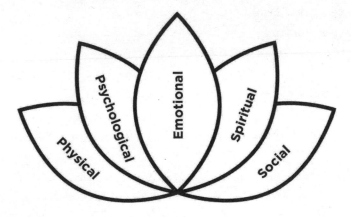

Feeling deserving of self-care is a significant task in itself, and something I would really encourage you to work on. If this feels totally alien to you, then you may need some support from close loved ones or from a qualified professional, who can help you to identify and work through your difficulties. Once you believe that you are deserving of self-love, then identifying self-care activities should come that bit more easily.

Physical – through our body

Physical self-care involves prioritising time to refuel your body so you can get on with living, moving and breathing. Here are my top ten tips:

1. Ask yourself: are you feeling hungry, angry, lonely or tired?
2. Build in regular exercise.
3. Eat healthily.
4. Get proper sleep.
5. Take pitstop naps.
6. Spend time outdoors.
7. Plan for screen-free time.
8. Have a good laugh.
9. Have some fun!
10. Try out the Headspace App.

Pause & reflect

What am I doing every day/week for my physical self-care?

_____

What I would like to do more of:

_____

Support I need to do it:

_____

Psychological – through our mind
Psychological self-care relates to nurturing positive mental health, a strong sense of self-compassion, and enriching your personal and professional development. Here are a few pointers:

1. Give attention to things that are within your control.
2. Take time for personal reflection.
3. Give up trying to stop negative thoughts – notice them, and let them go.
4. Schedule time to pursue an interest.
5. Try something new.
6. Step out of your comfort zone.
7. Build up your confidence.
8. Keep work and family life separate.
9. Follow the compassionate mind approach programme.[89]
10. Draw your three circles: see Compassion section, page 20.

Pause & reflect

What am I doing every day/week for my psychological self-care?

_____

What I would like to do more of:

_____

Support I need to do it:

_____

Emotional – through our heart
Emotional self-care relates to your ability to recognise your
feelings and to nurture the soothing part of your emotional
self. Here are a few pointers:

1. Explore both your own positive and negative feelings and
   what situations bring them up.
2. Learn how to say 'no'.
3. Reduce expectations on yourself; aim for good enough.
4. Choose who you spend time with.
5. Treat yourself!
6. Practise self-compassion and gently ease self-criticism.
7. Use positive and encouraging self-talk: 'I deserve my love.'
8. Share your feelings with someone else.
9. Be kind and help others. Consider volunteering.
10. Acknowledge childhood wounds and your shark music.
    Seek professional support if needed.

Pause & reflect

What am I doing every day/week for my emotional
self-care?

_____

What I would like to do more of:

_____

Support I need to do it:

_____

Spiritual – through our connection to something greater
Spiritual self-care is all about the essence of you as a human being in this present moment, and connecting to your purpose, finding meaning, and fostering creativity. Here are some pointers:

1. Determine your core values and what's most important to you in life.
2. Write down five things for which you are grateful each day.
3. Get some time alone.
4. Spend time in nature.
5. Make some time for self-reflection.
6. Get creative.
7. Cultivate calmness.
8. Recognise our common humanity.
9. Practise mindfulness and being in the present moment.
10. Try the **STOP** mindfulness exercise in the Appendices on page 251.

Pause & reflect

What am I doing every day/week for my spiritual self-care?

_____

What I would like to do more of:

_____

Support I need to do it:

_____

Social – through our connection with others
Social self-care relates to your ability to make and maintain
meaningful relationships, which is key to long-term emotional
and physical health. Here are a few pointers:

1. Enjoy emotional support.
2. Surround yourself with people who have got your back.
3. Seek out evidence-based advice – and balance it with what
   your gut tells you.
4. Accept practical support.
5. Nurture your relationships.
6. Choose your friends wisely.
7. Build in couple time.
8. Share the load: lower your expectations and ask for help.
9. Learn how to be assertive.
10. Get involved in your community.

Pause & reflect

What am I doing every day/week for my social self-care?

_____

What I would like to do more of:

_____

Support I need to do it:

_____

Anchoring

Holding tight, and letting go

> Growing up is a poorly choreographed dance: When you
> hold your child tight, they demand to be let go. When you
> let them go, they cry to be held tight.[90]

I really love the idea of the child–parent relationship being a
lifetime of experiences of holding tight and letting go, because
this captures the fine balance of parenting from the moment
of birth. When you first become a parent, nothing quite
prepares you for the all-consuming needs of your child, which
arise and fluctuate according to their stage of development
and their emerging sense of self.

> If we could look down from above and make a time-lapse
> video of parent and child spanning years, we'd see
> concentric circles. The setting would change from kitchen
> to bedroom to living room. From scouts to football
> practice to dance show. The child would grow and the
> parent would age. The clothes, the seasons and the years
> would all change, but the essential geometry would remain
> the same: child moves away from parent and then returns
> to centre. Away and back. Away and back. Further and
> further each time.
>
> The story is the same in infancy as the baby crawls
> away, looks around and then returns to centre. In primary
> school, the child discovers [friends and preferred
> activities]. In secondary school, the child explores groups,
> the internet and dating. The radius of those concentric
> circles centred around the anchor increases by magnitudes
> [as they gain more independence]. In young adulthood, the

child moves even further towards college, [travel] and work, friends and [partners]. Through it all, the anchor chain remains intact. Someday, perhaps, our kids will visit other planets but even then, measuring the radius of their movement in light years, the story will be the same. Holding tight and letting go.[91]

This dance of attunement shows the back-and-forth of every parent–child relationship since the beginning of time, the parent tuning in to their child and giving them the support and space they need until the child slowly gains their independence. In order for the child to develop healthily, they need to learn to draw on you as their safe haven during times of challenge, which will help them to rely on other loved ones as they grow older. Equally, they'll also need to learn to let go of you as their secure base,[92] and will need you to let go of them, which can be a really difficult thing to do for both parent and child.

Feeling the stress of the storm

In order to realise the worth of the anchor, we need to feel the stress of the storm.

Corrie ten Boom

These words resonate with many parts of me: the little girl who was always a little worrier and took the weight of the world on her shoulders; the parent who desperately wants to protect her daughters from the inevitable storms of life; and the clinical psychologist who helps parents like you to support their children through their stormy feelings.

An anxious child needs just this kind of anchor: an emotionally healthy parent who is solid and reliable, firm and constant, stable and secure; not perfect, but good enough, one who has weathered a few storms with their child. Your ability to anchor your child emotionally today enables them to feel secure and resilient tomorrow.

As your child's emotional anchor, you'll need your anchors to hold you steady too. As you'll know from your own life, finding out who your anchors are becomes clear in times of challenge. The same is true for your child.

When life is good and our needs are being met, when our environments feel safe and familiar, and when we feel secure in our close relationships, we feel free to let go and explore, learn and grow. We test our limits, and try out new ways of being and behaving. In the same way, when an anxious child feels safe, they'll allow themselves to float until they feel the tug of their anchor, and come back to replenish the sense of safety they need.

When your child feels threatened in any way by their environment or their own fearful thoughts, they're more likely to retreat closer to you as their emotional anchor and less likely to explore their world. It's like they're battening down the hatches for a storm. Whilst this shows their attachment towards you in seeking your comfort and support, there is a fine balance to be reached between holding tight and encouraging them to let go. In helping our children to feel anchored, we must also help them to feel safe being apart.

But how do we do this? Read on for my top tips for anchoring and cultivating safety.

You are my SAFE

Safe place
At five years of age
Things didn't seem quite right,
As you tossed and turned in bed
Before sitting up with a fright

The following morning
As the sun rose oh so high,
You clung to me fiercely
Refusing to say goodbye

Day after day
You would clutch your tummy tight,
Praying someone would notice
your internal fight

I am sorry all I saw
Was negative behaviour,
Especially as what you needed most
Was a guardian and saviour

You needed a safe place
Somewhere to call home,
A place to sink your anchor
Without fear of the unknown

But this storm you were hit with
It struck me too,
Knocking me off balance
With the dreaded fear of losing you

If I could go back in time
As you kicked and you screamed,
I'd pull you in closely
And remind you that you're everything I
 dreamed

I would tell you I can see your turmoil and
I'd tell you things will get better,
As from this day forward
We will take every step together

Caitriona McMahon

This captures so powerfully the idea of a parent's role as the child's emotional anchor during their stormy journey of anxiety.

Caitriona McMahon is a community mental health worker and co-founder of the Community Crisis Response Team in Limerick, Ireland. She has also worked as a swimming teacher to many fearful children over the years, which was her inspiration for writing this. Caitriona paints a picture of a five-year-old's fear of swimming, masked as a sore belly, poor sleep, fear of separation and negative behaviours. The poem also captures the parent's emotional distress at their child's suffering and the feeling of being powerless to help them, which hinders parents from seeing beyond their child's behaviour into their inner turmoil.

Caitriona sees her role as mediating between the child and the parent to increase the child's level of comfort and the parent's ability to support their child by being the child's safe place from where they can go out and test their fears. Caitriona works to unpack the child's worry by gently asking them questions related to how they're feeling. It's a process of elimination to figure out what specific aspect of swimming the child is struggling with.

Because it can sometimes take weeks for a child to immerse themselves in the water, Caitriona senses the parent's frustration at the pace of other children and things not moving more quickly. However, she feels that pressurising a child when they're already fearful will only make their fear worse. Furthermore, the child may pick up on their parent's frustration, which will make them feel less safe, as now the child feels that their parent isn't a safe place to go with their worry.

> Just imagine if you were around someone who freaked out
> when you freaked out. Wouldn't that make your panic so
> much worse? But when we are near someone who is able
> to stay calm in the midst of our panic, our body senses
> that it's okay to also rest and relax.[93]

A warm and attuned response from the parent provides the support and anchoring a child needs to understand, express and regulate their big feelings. Remaining calm in the midst of a child's panic facilitates them turning inwards, noticing what's happening inside their body, imagining their heart and breath slowing and their chest softening, and relating to themselves with kindness as they find the strength to ride through the fear.

If there's a message Caitriona most wants parents to hear in all her experience with fearful children over many years, it's the role parents play in helping their children with their big feelings rather than joining them in their distress:

> If I could go back in time as you kicked and you
>   screamed,
> I'd pull you in closely and remind you that you're
>   everything I dreamed.
> I'd tell you I can see your turmoil and I'd tell you
>   things will get better, as from this day forward
>   we'll take every step together.

This is what compassionate parenting is all about: slowing right down, seeing beyond negative behaviour to a child's inner turmoil, and letting them know you're there for them patiently every step along the way. It's about parents realising their crucial role in anchoring their child to safety whilst encouraging their gradual exposure to the things they fear. It's about using a child's future anxious moments to encourage them to become their own safe place in years to come.

A case in point: Andrew

Andrew, aged seven, came to the pool on his second week of lessons crippled with fear, holding on to his belly and his mummy for dear life. As he hadn't been afraid the previous week, Caitriona put on her detective hat and unpacked his worry a little: 'Is there any particular stroke that you do that makes the pain in your belly worse?' she asked.

By relating the question to his very real physical experience, Caitriona validated Andrew's feelings without any judgement. Asking the question in a calm and genuinely interested way also gave her the best chance of understanding what was wrong.

'When I swim backwards I keep thinking that I'm going to drown – but I know that I'm not,' Andrew replied.

Caitriona was captivated. Although Andrew's body insisted there was a threat, he had the wisdom to realise that reality didn't match his fears.

'I'm not going to force you to do anything you don't want to do,' she said. 'After a while we could try it, and if you don't feel comfortable just put up your hand and we'll stop practising that stroke for today.'

This worked well. It's all about patience, calmness and giving the control back to the child, setting the foundation from which they're better able to build the confidence to face their fears in their own way and at their own pace. Caitriona finds that the kids who take their time to begin with are the very ones who now absolutely love swimming!

. . . .

How to manage separations
Another common time for everyday anxiety to appear for children is when they're separated from their parents, whether for short or longer periods of time. No matter what the length of the separation, not managing it well can actually lead to greater anxiety for a child. Here we'll go through what managing separations well actually looks like.

It's crucial for parents to keep their child informed of impending separations, especially a child with anxiety. This may include everything from a parent going to the shop, to a minder picking up children from school instead of a parent, to a night away at Granny's, to a business trip or a parent going into hospital. Although separations are very difficult for many kids, they're a necessary part of life and something that we can learn to navigate in the smoothest possible way.

There seems to be a myth that less information about separation will protect children from their feelings of distress. Not so. Too little information fuels anxiety because it can weaken the trust between a child and their parent.

Imagine if one minute your safety net was in sight, and the next it was gone. Saying 'Goodbye' and explaining the plan allows your child to air their feelings within your calm and comforting presence so they can move on to exploring their environment without you. Security provides the foundation for this exploration. Without it, a child is left to manage their big feelings on their own.

The 'Goodbye' for anxious children can be a long and drawn-out process, which many parents report can be distressing for everyone involved. No wonder it may seem easier for parents not to go out or to keep children away from things they fear, or to nip out quickly, hoping not to be noticed!

But delaying the inevitable won't help an anxious child in the long run. Children need to be separated from you on occasion, but they need to feel some level of control and safety within that. This is done by telling them what is happening: where you're going, who will be looking after them and what they may be doing while you're away, and approximately when you expect to be back.

If your child has a tendency to contact you a lot when you're out, cap the number of times they can contact you, as reassurance keeps anxiety alive. For example, say: 'You can only ring me X times when I'm out. You'll be having loads of fun with your aunt and can talk to her if you need.' Reduce the number of times they can contact you as you practise going out more.

Another thing to consider is that your child may sense your discomfort in letting them go, as you may fear for their safety or well-being. Anxious kids sniff out parental worries in an instant! For this reason, parents may also need to manage their own anxiety around separations. It's a delicate balance … one that can be fraught with difficulty, but which brings opportunities to improve things for you and your child if handled with care.

A case in point: Milly

There is an old school of thought that supports a child being distracted while the parent quickly ducks out of sight when leaving them. Result: less stress for parent, less trust for child.

A mother came to see me about her 'clingy' six-year-old daughter Milly, who found separations from her upsetting. I asked Mum about who was looking after Milly today and how Milly had taken to Mum leaving. Mum said that Milly's older sibling was taking care of her and that 'I slipped out of the house without saying anything to avoid a big scene.'

I totally get where Milly's mother was coming from. Her intentions were good in trying to protect her daughter from upset, without knowing that this choice could actually be causing distrust. So I asked, 'How do you think Milly might feel when she knows you've left?' Mum said she wasn't sure and hoped she would be all right.

I told Mum that I appreciated how difficult this was for both of them, then helped her to see it from Milly's perspective: 'If you leave without saying anything, Milly may well imagine the worst. Although her brother's there, she doesn't have you to soothe her big feelings. This could make her trust you less, so she'll be damn sure not to let you leave her side again in future.'

Another aspect I needed to bring to Mum's attention was the possibility that Milly was finding it difficult to separate from her mother as she was worried about *her mother's* emotional well-being. Milly's mother suffered from periods of low mood, which it was likely Milly had picked up on, even if these were outside of her conscious awareness. The idea that Milly might be concerned for her mother's well-being was news to Mum, so we took this into account as we explored how separations could be managed in future.

If you have a child with separation anxiety, it might be worth asking yourself:

- 'Is there anything going on in my life that may concern my child about my well-being?'
- 'How do I feel about my child separating from me and going into the outside world?'
- 'When my child resists separating from me, how do I feel in the moment and how might this be coming across to my child?'

And finally:

- 'Is there any way that I can anchor my child during our separations?'

This brings to mind a beautiful storybook I often read to my children called *The Invisible String* by Patrice Karst. The mother in the story introduces the idea to soothe her fearful twins:

> People who love each other are always connected by a very special String made of love. Even though you can't see it with your eyes, you can feel it deep in your heart and know that you're always connected to the ones you love. When you're at school and you miss me, your love travels all the way along the String until I feel it tug on my heart.[94]

Isn't that just beautiful? This is what anchoring your child is all about: letting them know that no matter how wide the physical distance is between you, they're 'kept in mind' within their nurturing relationship with you. My girls just love this,

as do I, and it certainly makes those necessary separations
that bit easier.

Top tips for anchoring and cultivating safety

Not only are you your child's emotional anchor – you're also
their safe place to fall so they can let go of their fears. This
brings to mind the incredible courage shown by trapeze artists
performing in a circus, testing themselves to the limit knowing that their firm and supportive safety net will catch them if
they fall. Similarly, in building your child's sense of safety,
you're that net that enables them to take risks so that their
edges of tolerance can be tested.

Children have a greater capacity to seek support from their
parents and to benefit from it when their nervous system feels
safe. By contrast, they have more need to fight, flee or freeze
when their nervous system senses danger. This is why it's
important to take steps to consciously cultivate your child's
sense of safety and to anchor their anxiety.

Do a self-check first

What constitutes safety in a child's environment are the subtle
safety cues from those closest to them. These might include
your facial expression, the tone of your voice and the calmness
in your body. It's less *what* you say but *how* you show your
genuine affection for them. It may be difficult for your child
to switch into safe mode unless you feel calm from the inside
out, which is where a self-check list comes in.

As parents, when we interact with children who are emotionally unregulated, it's natural to feel distressed. Working on
nurturing calm from the inside out involves a deeper exploration
of how you respond to your child's anxiety and whether your
shark music impacts in any way. When you're in contact with
your child during their most anxious moments, ask yourself:

- What is happening inside my nervous system?
- Are my coping skills activated?
- What tone of voice am I using?
- What is my body language communicating?
- Do I feel safe right now?

Cultivating safety to mirror calm and containment is a tall order when your child is midway through an anxiety attack. In those incredibly tough moments, use your compassionate voice to answer the following:

- What do I need right now to feel safe?
- Do I need to take a deep breath, to take five, or to call someone to help me?

Managing yourself is really challenging, but it is also an opportunity to provide valuable modelling for your child. Taking the time to build on your connection, including awareness of your child's sense of safety and your shark music, builds a solid foundation from which they can begin to feel safe in testing out their edges of tolerance, so they can learn and grow from them.

It's about finding the sweet spot where you encourage your child to move ever so slightly outside their comfort zone and hold them safe if they fall. This could take a bit of practice. To help you on your way, here are my top tips on how to cultivate safety for your anxious child. They can also be used by any support person, including a family member, educator or friend.

The Fear-O-Meter

For younger children, I really recommend using a feelings thermometer or a 'Fear-O-Meter'[95] for tuning in to your child's inner experience. Choose a time when you're both relaxed. All you need is paper and markers or pencils. Draw a thermome-ter with a scale from 0 to 10, where 0 is 'easy peasy' (happy face), 6 is 'getting tough' (uneasy face) and 10 is 'out of control' (freaked-out face). Try colour-coding it from green at the bottom, to orange in the middle, to red at the top. Let your child take the lead in labelling their Fear-O-Meter using words or pictures they like.

- The Fear-O-Meter will give you and your child a way to talk about anxiety both when they're calm and when they're anxious.
- By rating their own subjective experience, your child learns what makes them anxious, and you both get a sense of how calm or distressed they feel at any given moment.
- Choosing a number on their Fear-O-Meter engages your child's mind, and makes them stop and focus. This makes it much harder for them to remain anxious, as their brain is otherwise occupied.
- The Fear-O-Meter is a tool to measure changes in anxiety, up or down, which can help you to decide which anxiety-management techniques work best for your child.

Relaxation and stress-reduction techniques

In taking action together with your child to work through some of their anxiety, I would encourage you to try out some of these tried-and-tested techniques listed here and in the appendices, and see which works best. The aim is to connect with your child by helping them to release built-up tension through physical activity – relaxation, play and physical touch – which will help to ground them, shift their fearful thoughts and improve their sense of control.[96]

- *Ice-cold Water* – When a child is in fight-flight-freeze mode, they need your soothing and help to become 'unscared'. Making sure to get their permission first, splash drops of really cold water on their temples to slow their heart rate and turn the panic right down.
- *Shaking on Purpose* – This can be used to meet a child's high energy in fight-flight-freeze mode or to help a child recover from being in frozen mode. Get them to jump up and down, scream or make noises and make their whole bodies shake. Do it with them so they won't feel so self-conscious. Because fight-flight-freeze blocks their natural expression of fear, Shaking on Purpose helps children to let some of their feelings out in a safe way.
- *Butterfly Hug*[97] – Try this yourself first, then show your child. Cross your arms in front of you and pat your shoulders, alternating right- and left-handed pats. Alternate gentle squeezes of each shoulder. Add on by visualising a safe place or silently repeating a word or phrase that represents security (e.g. 'I'm safe' or 'Peace'). Alternating between left and right reduces anxiety as it activates both sides of the brain. Comforting touch also releases oxytocin, which helps disperse high cortisol levels, bringing your child back to a calmer state.
- *The 5–4–3–2–1 Game* – This a great technique for anchoring children to the here and now, using their senses during panicky moments. Best practised when calm.

1. Describe five things you see in the room.
2. Name four things you can feel, e.g. 'my feet on the floor' or 'the air in my nose'.
3. Name three things you hear, e.g. 'traffic outside'.
4. Name two things you can smell, or two smells you like.
5. Name one good thing about yourself.

- *Figure-8 Breathing* – Anxious children often use this exercise on their own, quietly and privately wherever they are (even in class!). Ask your child to imagine their index finger as a pencil drawing a figure 8 on their skin or using their big toe to draw a figure 8 on the ground. As they're drawing the first half of the figure 8, breathe in for three. When they get to the middle, hold their finger still for one. Then, for the second half of the figure 8, breathe out for three. When they get to the middle, hold for one again. Repeat three or four times. Parents, feel free to practise this at home.[98]
- *The Tunnel*[99] – Ask your child to draw a tunnel. If you were ever to become anxious driving through a tunnel, the best option is usually to keep going rather than to go back. When your child is anxious, ask them to imagine passing through the tunnel repeating the words, 'This feeling will pass.'
- *Counting Down* – One of the simplest techniques is asking your child their number on the Fear-O-Meter and counting down slowly from that number down to one. When they're finished, ask them for their new number, which hopefully will be a little lower. If not, repeat or count down, with them visualising walking down a staircase. You could add words between each number (e.g. '7, more and more relaxed, 6, more and more relaxed …').
- *Dragon Fire Breath* – Ask your child to link their fingers under their chin, inhale a big dragon breath through their nose and lift their elbows up to frame their face. Exhale, lifting their head up and opening their mouth wide to make a 'Hah' sound towards the sky like a dragon blowing fire. Lower the elbows back down to meet at the bottom by the end of the 'Hah' sound. This is a good energising technique that helps to build confidence.
- *Rhythmic Activity* – The key to using exercise to relieve anxiety is to work the body hard using rhythmic activity like running or jumping jacks. Trying exercises together first is best.

- *Heartbeat Exercise* – Children are timed doing jumping jacks for 30 seconds, then asked to lie down and place their hand on their heart, relax, breathe deeply and feel their heartbeat slowing down.
- *The Bounce* – Children stand and bounce gently up and down on the balls of their feet, where their heels rise and fall, never touching the ground. They can add a little shake of their hands if they like, as if they're shaking off water.
- *Sensory Activity* – Engaging a child's senses is a great way to release anxious tension. When they're feeling anxious, get your child to do something as simple as pouring liquid between containers over and over again. Have a try at the Slime and Glitter Jar activities when you're both feeling calm. These can then be used when your child is feeling anxious.

Slime!

Most children who come to see me also adore making slime, because it really relaxes them and they end up sharing a lot with me during the production process! I know not every parent is comfortable with slime, but it can be made without too much fuss:

- Pour a small cup (30 ml) of PVA glue into a bowl.
- Add a few drops of food colouring or paint (not strictly necessary) and stir.
- Slowly add 1 teaspoon of liquid laundry detergent. Mix all together.
- Pick up and stretch and fold in your hands until it becomes less sticky and more slime-like.
- Conserve in a container. If it becomes sticky again, add a small dash of laundry detergent.
- Enjoy! Your kids will love you for it!

Glitter jars

Making these together is another favourite for children and parents alike:

- Use an empty glass jar or water bottle and fill it with water and glitter.
- Add food colouring or glitter glue for colour if you like.
- Close the jar firmly with the lid and shake it.
- During an anxious moment, say to your child, 'All the glitter exploding is your thoughts and feelings right now. Let's breathe deeply together and watch the glitter settle.'
- Practise controlled breathing: 'Inhale for a count of 4 (1–2–3–4), hold for a count of 4 (1–2–3–4), and exhale for a count of 4 (1–2–3–4).'

- *Yoga Poses* – There are a number of yoga poses parents like to use that promote relaxation. For The Mountain pose, ask your child to:

1. Stand with back straight, look straight ahead or close their eyes, arms by their side.
2. Imagine the crown of their head lifting upward, as their feet remain firmly planted.
3. Try it first in shoes, then barefoot to increase awareness of the solid ground under their feet.

While your child is in The Mountain pose, a variation is The Challenge:

1. Tell your child you're going to give them a little push against their side (not too hard!).
2. For the first go, ask them to think about something that makes them anxious, then push. You'll probably notice that they're easily pushed off balance.
3. Have your child think about being a mountain, anchored to the bedrock of the earth, with lots of inner strength and resources.
4. Give the same push and see if they stay a little steadier this time, maybe swaying a little but not losing balance.
5. Have them think about the difference in their bodies between the off-balance feeling of anxiety and the power of feeling anchored.

A fun variation of this is for you as parent to be the mountain, while your child is a strong storm trying to knock you over! Hold your ground for a while, then fall over in a funny way.

- *My Hands Are Heavy and Warm* – This is a nice physical-touch exercise to do with your child:

1. Get comfortable together, close your eyes and take your child's hands in yours.
2. Gently say, 'My hands are heavy and warm,' and keep repeating this for a couple of minutes.
3. Most children feel a heavy, warm or tingly feeling as a result of the increased blood flow to the extremities, taking the blood away from the anxiety centres of the gut and chest.

- *Safe Place Guided Imagery* – Most children have good imaginations, so painting a relaxing picture with words, focusing on their safe place, works well. Ask them to imagine lying on a beach, walking in the woods, floating on a cloud, or whatever feels safe to them, and develop a story that ends with the words: 'Your safe place is there for you whenever you need.'

 For further and play-based exercises, flip ahead to the Appendices, page 241 to find the right one for you and your child.

Feeling felt

The secret message

The third step in the SAFE Chain of Resilience after self-care and anchoring is helping your child to feel felt. Feeling felt is all about relating to your child, and helping them to feel calm and contained. By helping children feel felt, our goal is for them to know that they have our support, and assist them in developing the capacity to regulate their own emotions by learning from our example. This enables them to use the parts of their brain that allow for true connection and rational reasoning.

Feeling felt means feeling understood, and it has an incredible impact. Feeling like someone 'gets' us is one of our most primal human needs, without which we end up feeling lost. Feeling felt is especially meaningful for children whose emotions can be chaotic at times, as they fully rely on us as their caregivers to provide safety, acceptance and guidance:

> When we attune to others we allow our own internal state
> to shift, to come to resonate with the inner world of
> another. This resonance is at the heart of the important
> sense of 'feeling felt' that emerges in close relationships.
> Children need attunement to feel secure and to develop
> well, and throughout our lives we need attunement to feel
> close and connected.[100]

In our modern world, with so much focus on 'doing', feeling felt helps children look inwards, where their vulnerabilities are, but also from where their kindness and resilience grow:

> The truth is, rarely can a response make something better
> – what makes something better is connection. And that
> connection requires mutual vulnerability … To feel is to
> be vulnerable.[101]

Helping children make sense of their mixed-up emotions requires an empathetic response from parents. This can often make parents feel vulnerable, because in order for a parent to connect with their child's big feeling, they need to connect with something inside themselves that knows the feeling.[102] This is understandably difficult for parents whose shark music is playing loud and strong. This recognition is key in how you respond.

A really valuable way to actively tune in to your child is to focus on the need behind your child's behaviour: what are they trying to tell you through their behaviour? That is the 'secret message' behind their anxiety. It can be helpful to ask yourself:

If my child's distress could speak, I wonder what would it say?

If my child's fears or worries had a message, what would it be?

Thinking of our child struggling to handle something difficult encourages us to help them through their big feelings. A common obstacle preventing parents from doing this is when they judge whether their child has a good enough reason to be feeling what they're feeling or not.

You know you're doing it when you start a sentence with, 'But that shouldn't be bothering you', 'It'll be fine, don't worry about it' or even 'This is ridiculous' (that was me last night). It can be really hard to empathise sometimes, because children's feelings fluctuate like crazy and sometimes don't make a lot of sense (e.g. broken bananas, anyone?!). When this happens, our default setting can be to judge.

But judging your child's feelings inevitably backfires, as they're left with a feeling that *feels* real to them, with no one to make sense of it with them. It's important to remember that children cannot reason like you or me, and that they don't have our experience of life's rollercoaster of emotions. No matter how nonsensical, frustrating or frightening our children's feelings may appear to us, they're real and important to them, and we need to bear this in mind when we consider how to respond.

> If your child's distress could speak, perhaps you'd hear it say:
>
> • I need you to be with me in this really tough moment.
> • I'm struggling with a really scary feeling.
> • I'm so afraid and confused. I need you to anchor me to safety.
> • Help, I don't know how to make it better by myself.
> • Stay with me in my messy feeling.
> • Let's breathe in and out of it together.
> • Try not to judge or minimise it.
> • Try not to rationalise or problem-solve it.
> • Gently guide me through it. Please don't push, as I'll get there in the end!
> • You are my one and only. I need you more than you think.
> • If not you, then who?

Validation of feelings

Taking your child's distress seriously and acknowledging what is happening as being very real for them helps them hugely, and is good practice for building their own ability to empathise with others. Validation of feelings is an essential component of positive mental health for children because it gives them an experience of being safe and connected as they learn about their feelings and helps them feel felt. It's all about the parents' capacity to understand and share their children's big feelings, such as sadness, joy, anger, curiosity, pain, frustration or excitement.

It's equally important that the parents' own feelings be validated. This is something that they may not have experienced when they were children, which can make it harder for them to see the need behind their child's behaviour.

Think about how you feel towards your child when they express anxiety; we don't all have good feelings towards our children all of the time, *and that is OK!* It's as if they live in a different universe sometimes. They can press our buttons, making it hard to meet their needs, *and that is OK!* The important thing is to acknowledge your own feelings when this happens, and to find the strength you have within to ride the wave and delay reacting until you're in a better way. By doing this, you can build your relationship with them and help develop their emotional regulation.

'If not you, then who?' has been thought provoking for me both as a mum and as a psychologist. Parents are under a lot of pressure to 'do, do, do' all the time, trying to meet a lot of high expectations and extrinsic goals. But if not you, then who will sit quietly with your child, look into their eyes and listen to them intently? If not you, then who will hold them close and let them know everything's going to be OK?

Connect and redirect[103]

Our emotions spring from the right side of the brain, and reason springs from the left side.

When a child is overwhelmed by emotion, it's the right side of their brain that's doing the talking – or crying or shouting! Because a child's anxiety can trigger discomfort in the parent, a parent's reaction can be to smooth it over quickly, to judge the feeling, minimise it or try to solve it like they would any other problem. These are all left-brained responses, which unfortunately miss the mark.

Here's why: the child's right side cannot process information from the parent's left side, so your reasoning and logic won't work.

> When a child is upset, logic often won't work until we have responded to the right brain's emotional needs. We call this emotional connection 'attunement', which is how we connect deeply with another person and allow them to 'feel felt'.[104]

Here's an example:

> Child in right-brained (emotional) distress: *'I'm so worried a monster could come into my room!'*

> Parent's left-brain (reasoned) response: *'Don't be silly, monsters don't exist. You'll be fine once you close your eyes. No more scary films for you. Go to sleep now and stop thinking about that!'*

In our society, where we're trained to work things out using words and logic, it's news to most parents that logic is of little use when their child is deeply distressed.

Instead, the parent can use the emotional right side of their brain to connect with their child. By reacting in a calm and soothing way, the parent appeals to the emotional right side of the child's brain. Acknowledge their feelings, and use physical touch, empathetic facial expressions, a nurturing tone of voice and listen without judging.

> Parent's right-brain (emotional) response: *'You seem worried about the idea of monsters coming into your room. Worries can be really tough can't they and feel big, especially at night-time. You are safe, darling. Why don't I stay here with you and we can cuddle and relax until you're ready for me to go, then tomorrow we can talk a bit more about how to make your worry less scary?'*

This right-to-right brain connection allows you to communicate with your distressed child. It's in this calmer state that being physically close to your child – be it touching them gently, putting your arm around them, holding their hand, whatever they feel comfortable with – also helps to give them that all-important shot of the bonding hormone oxytocin.

It's only when the parent has helped their child to feel felt in this way that it becomes possible to redirect the conversation with logic and reason, appealing to the child's left brain using the parent's left brain. This is done by talking logically with a child about their feelings, thoughts and behaviours when they're in a better place to do so, either later on or the following day. Using humour can also help in 'silly-fying' the fear.

 Flip ahead to 'A case in point: silly-fying the fear' (page 206), which can help when working through these ideas with your children.

Anxiety made simple

HALT and think: are they Hungry, Angry, Lonely or Tired?

As parents will recognise, there are times when a child has simply gone past the point of no return, when connect and redirect may not work as well.

In these moments, a child may be Hungry, Angry, Lonely or Tired (HALT), and will benefit from their basic needs being met first. During these times, address and try to maintain that soothing connection with your child. Anchoring techniques work best here. Calm them down, address their basic needs, and go back to the connect and redirect strategy when they're more responsive to it: 'I'd like to talk about this again after we've all had a good night's sleep.'

Talking about your child's feelings

> We are wired to feel safest and bravest when we are
> connected to our favourite humans.[105]

Your child's emotional brain is also designed to recruit support from someone who understands. One of the best ways to let your child know that you're there for them is to name your child's feelings to show them that you understand (e.g. 'You seem worried about the test tomorrow'). You can also ask your child to name their own feeling, which again helps to make them stop, focus and use both sides of their brain.

Talking about the feeling normalises it, and can give you an opportunity to tell them that emotions are like waves – they come and they go, and while your child might feel like this now, they'll not feel this way forever. It helps them to understand that their feelings are common to us all and there's no shame in having any of them. Reminding them to bring kindness to their feelings can also bring relief.

> Although we can't control the messages our children face when they're at school or with friends, we can cultivate a place where emotions are heard and validated at home, by using the language of feelings.
>
> Talk about your child's feelings and how you manage your own feelings too: 'I felt angry about that, but taking a breath helped me to calm down.' Children of parents who use the language of feelings are better able to express and name their feelings, which is an invaluable tool for coping with anxiety.

Tough times build attachment

Children develop a secure attachment to their parent when the parent is sensitive to their signals and responds appropriately to their needs, which happens naturally *some of the time*. The rest of the time, a sense of attachment is built in the aftermath of problems. This is what good enough parenting is all about.[106]

After all, being attuned to your child's needs and making sure they feel felt is not something a parent can do for their child every time something is amiss. Don't worry, we're all in the same boat. There are many reasons preventing us from connecting to one another, including fear of pain, tiredness, impatience, anger, frustration, apathy, distraction, ignorance or getting caught up in our own lives.

Relationship ruptures or setbacks are common and result from the challenges when a parent and child read and respond to each other's cues. For example, if a parent is feeling overwhelmed at a particular moment, or if the child is expressing themselves in a challenging way, they're less able to read their child's need and more likely to see their *child* as the problem. We've all been there!

Ruptures can also happen when a parent feels powerless in the face of their child's anxiety. Because anxiety is contagious, a child's alarmed state can make it difficult for parents to remain calm. An anxious child may also misread cues when grappling with an overactive fight-flight-freeze response. No matter how well intentioned a parent might be, this may impair the child's ability to receive comfort and security.

It's no wonder ruptures happen so often, but if a parent can take a step back, it can be a precious opportunity to repair the relationship. Parents of securely attached children are more likely to see a rupture as part of the natural course of parenting and as one of those 'survive-and-thrive'[107] moments that can serve to strengthen their relationship with their child.

Now for the fluffy feel-good bit. *Relationship repairs are transformative.* There is a great beauty in repairing a rupture, although parents may not realise this, which might be traced back to the era of authoritarian parenting styles, when apologising to a child would have seemed outrageous. So have I got news for you. *Repair* is the fertile ground upon which you can teach your child many valuable life lessons, like what it means to be human, to make mistakes, to try to make amends, and to associate a rupture with the hope and possibility of a repair. You can acknowledge your own mistakes and apologise – teaching them by example – which they'll then learn to do themselves in their relationships with you and with others. Repair builds a healthy pathway in your child's brain – they'll come to expect support following stress, which will encourage them to seek out healthy relationships as they grow older.

For example, there is huge power in calmly explaining to your child: 'I'm sorry for how I spoke to you earlier. That wasn't OK. My feelings felt very big at the time and I'm guessing that didn't feel nice for you. Taking a deep breath and resetting my brain would have helped me to understand you better. Can we try again?'

It's important to note that saying 'I'm sorry' followed by blame doesn't count. 'I'm sorry for how I spoke to you, but what you did made me so frustrated!' will push your child away and will not repair your relationship. Explain, be calm and leave it at that for the moment. If there's a lesson to be learned from the situation, go back to it again when you're both feeling calm and connected together: 'I'm sorry for over-reacting earlier. Next time we could both try one of our anchoring techniques to help us find a good way forward together.'

Decades of attachment research shows us that attuning to children's needs and being with them in their big feelings helps them to feel less overwhelmed and more secure. Feeling felt, understanding that feelings are transient and can be survived, and learning that there is light at the end of the emotional tunnel enables a child to build trust in you and the world. It also shows them how to regulate their emotions, to attune to others and builds their empathy and resilience.

Storytelling: helping younger children feel felt

When a child is helped to think about his troubled feelings through story, it can prevent these feelings from building up into an awful mess inside. In other words, used well, stories can become a vital part of a child's healthy emotional digestive system.[108]

When very young children are struggling with difficult new feelings, they can show up as nightmares, fears, bedwetting, poor sleep and so on. Just like food, children's painful feelings need to be properly digested and worked through. Because little children do not talk naturally or easily about their feelings, they can end up bottling them up, which is precisely why their feelings leak out in other ways.

Very often, children under the age of eight or so do not manage their big feelings very well, nor do they have the inner resources to think their problems through or problem-solve. For this reason, parents need a way of communicating with young children using *their* language, in order to help them feel understood and validated.

Humans have been telling stories since the beginning of time. Storytelling is how we connect with one another, it's how we find meaning, laugh, cry and heal. Because memories and emotions spring from the right side of our brains, while the factual details of our lives reside in the left, storytelling helps us to make sense of an event using our whole brain, which is the best way to process something difficult and to heal from it.

Ask your child to tell their own story

When a child is afraid, the right side of their brain is automatically in charge. This can lead to worst-case-scenario thinking: 'I saw someone get bitten by a dog. All dogs bite people.' Once a child has been anchored and calmed by their parent, encouraging them to tell the story of what they're afraid of can be very powerful in opening them up to logic.

Sometimes parents avoid talking about upsetting experiences, thinking that doing so will reinforce their children's pain or make things worse. Actually, telling the story is often exactly what children need, both to make sense of the event and to move on to a place where they can feel better about what happened.[109]

If your child is afraid of dogs, it could be useful to ask them the story of the first time they remember being scared by a dog. To tell a story that makes sense, they must engage both sides of their brain. The right side gives them access to the bodily sensations, raw emotions and personal memories; the left side puts things in order using words and logic. Once their left-brain logic is working alongside their right-brain emotions to make sense of their initial scary experience, their response to the next dog they see might tend towards, 'This dog is OK because it looks calmer and people are petting it. My parents told me that it's a friendly dog.'[110]

Read a storybook together

There are times when children won't want to tell their stories when we ask them to. This is perfectly understandable, and we need to respect their wishes about *how* and *when* to talk. A great way to engage them is by reading them a therapeutic story, one that speaks about the problem they're having. A therapeutic story speaks of common emotional issues, like worries and fears, but does so using the power of the imagination.

In another favourite story of mine, *Teenie Weenie in a Too Big World*,[111] a tiny creature, Teenie Weenie, finds himself in a place full of noises and things that swoop and scratch. The worse it gets, the smaller he feels, so small indeed that the tiniest insect tries to eat him up, leaving him feeling terrified and desperately alone. Along strolls a Wip-Wop bird, who invites him into his treehouse for a chocolate muffin. With his new friend, Teenie Weenie learns about the power of being together, and so when he's struggling alone he finds someone to help him.

Therapeutic stories like this work really well because they provide the distance a child often needs from their own painful story. Carefully chosen for a particular issue, a therapeutic story can give you special access into a child's inner world. While the story is being read, a child is likely to identify with the main character, will experience the character's obstacles but also feel the character's courage to overcome them. After hearing the story, the child will have two pictures of the painful situation: the old picture, pre-story, and the new picture, post-story, enriched by all the empathy, wisdom and creative possibility the tale has provided.[112]

Paint a picture
Other ways of using storytelling to connect with your child include asking them to tell you a story through painting or colouring (i.e. 'Can you show me what your fear looks like?'). Or you could try sharing with them a story about a fear you had when you were a child and how you managed it, by drawing it out for them. This helps children to see that they're not alone in having fears, which comes as such a relief to them.

Remote of the mind
For older children, I find the 'remote of the mind' technique works really well. Children often shy away from replaying bad or scary memories following a difficult event, but it's important for them to understand the importance of exploring what has happened to them.

Gently encourage your child to tell the story back using their internal remote control, where they can pause when they need a break, fast-forward through scary parts until they're ready, and rewind and replay the story again as often as they need to. Make sure to end up telling the entire story at some point, even the scary parts. In this way, children can maintain control over how much of the story they view.[113]

Techniques like storytelling and unpacking a worry are a bridge between the feeling felt and empowerment steps, as they fulfil your child's need to feel connected and understood so they are free to move on to a calmer place of empowerment and learning.

Empowerment

Wisdom is not found in the feeling brain (limbic system)
or the thinking brain (prefrontal cortex) but in the
dialogue between the two.[114]

The final step of the SAFE Chain of Resilience is empowerment, which refers to parents enabling their child to take
control of their anxiety by arming them with a coping toolkit.
At the core of a child's well-being is the integration of separate
areas of the brain, which enables insight, empathy, kindness
and resilience.[115]

It's only when a child's core needs have been met (i.e. self-
care, anchoring and feeling felt) that they're in a position to
welcome and implement anxiety-management techniques
using their reasoning brains.

In this section we'll look at three powerful ways of managing
anxiety. The first is play, which is the perfect antidote to
children's anxiety up to the teenage years. The second is
cognitive behavioural therapy (CBT), which looks at the
relationship between children's thoughts, feelings and
behaviours and teaches young people (i.e. aged eight and up)
everyday skills to manage anxiety. And finally, mindfulness
meets kindfulness, which promotes the integration of the
brain and is key to lifelong resilience for children of all ages.

Playing with anxiety

For a child it is in the simplicity of play that the
complexity of life is sorted like puzzle pieces joined
together to make sense of the world.

L. R. Knost

There truly is a magic and a healing in play. I couldn't have written a book on children's anxiety without exploring its rich rewards, which I've witnessed with many little children ... and big children – their parents!

Play is a child's bread and butter. It's not an optional part of children's lives, but is absolutely crucial for every aspect of their physical, emotional, social and cognitive development. Play guides children's development, and they can be trusted to choose the right kind of play for that moment in their development.

> Because play is a child's language and toys are their words,[116] it follows that in order for adults to best communicate with children, playing with them and having playful interactions is key.

As mentioned before, children's anxiety can be further compounded by adults' difficulties in understanding or responding effectively to what they're feeling and trying to communicate to us. This communication gap can be widened when adults expect children to talk through their feelings, which they may not yet have the verbal skills to do. This is why play is to a child what words are to an adult. Just like talking about your worries with a close loved one will usually make you feel better, play does the same for children as it's their natural medium for expression.

Of course, play also happens to be the perfect antidote to children's – and their parents' – anxiety thanks to the fun, enjoyment and pleasure it brings.[117] Whatever your age, you simply cannot feel anxious when you're immersed in playing. Play brings laughter and laughter loosens fear.[118] Play brings a child calmness and a sense of control over their world, which help them to feel safe in their most challenging moments. Playful techniques can be used by parents to anchor their anxious child back to safety, helping them to feel loved and opening them up to reason.

Children need the opportunity to play with you as their parent and to play freely with other children. Most anxious children benefit from playful strategies in calming them down, while some also benefit from play therapy with a qualified practitioner.

Parent–child play

> If a child is to keep alive his inborn sense of wonder, he needs the companionship of at least one adult who can share it ... rediscovering with him the joy, excitement, and mystery of the world we live in.
>
> *Rachel Carson*

You may not realise it but your child is your biggest fan. They adore you and look up to you – and what wouldn't they do to spend some quality time with you. Because play is children's most natural form of expression, they're most likely to respond to us as parents if we communicate and connect with them using play.

Play is a powerful tool to deepen your connection and to bring your child to a place of safety and calm. Children have a deep need to feel delighted in, which builds the foundations for their self-esteem and fosters their sense of belonging.

Playing with your child helps them to feel special. Rather than focus on their worries, it gives you and your child a chance to spend some valuable time together and reduces some of the tension that accompanies anxiety. Child–parent play also lays the foundation for working through challenges together.

Sadly, I've noticed that child–parent play can sometimes be seen as an added luxury in a busy household, rather than as something that both young and old really need to nurture family connections. I know we're all busy, and both parents often have to work to make ends meet, so setting aside time to play with your child or to be playful can be a real challenge.

As a mum, psychologist, wife, and now author, I wonder where the time is going to come from. I often feel guilty coming home from a day playing with other people's kids that I can't be more energetic for my own. My girlies look at me with their sad expressions, asking for their 'Mammy time', which they're perfectly entitled to after a day away from me. So I tell them that they'll get their time after food and pyjamas. Whether it's playing a game, chilling out reading a story or just acting silly, we all get a chance to reconnect after a long day. I find it helpful to put a time limit on it as my energy and reserves of patience can be low, to say the least! FYI, I don't manage 'Mammy time' every day, but I try to at least a few times a week.

A short blast of quality time with parents gives children the chance to counterbalance the negative feelings they can carry around with them all day, including anxious thoughts. Consider this special play time as refilling your child's emotional cup so they can go back to exploring their world full-up with love and possibility.[119]

What I generally recommend is that parents set aside ten minutes or so each day for special play time with their children. If this isn't feasible, I would recommend that you prioritise this at least three times a week. Build it into your routine in a way that's not overwhelming for you. Taking small opportunities to be playful and silly throughout the day is also recommended because it connects you back to yourself and your relationship.

Playing with your kids and being playful can also be really enjoyable and fun! Kids just love seeing their parents smiling and being in the moment with them. There's nothing like a good auld tickle, a crazy dance around the kitchen or a competitive board game to bring out the child in everyone. It's all about purposefully creating a space in which to relax and to forget – if only for a few minutes – about the routines that can wear us all down.

Being playful in how you ask questions encourages children to express themselves more freely. When asked 'how was your day?', children often give one-word answers. Instead ask them about the best bit and least best bit of their day, which is sure to bring you richer detail. My girls also love to play 'Tell me two truths and one lie about today and I'll guess the lie.' We can all end up getting quite creative!

Parents of older children may think their kids are too old to play. There are always ways to be playful and to spend quality time with a child of any age. A child is never too old to feel delighted in and to benefit from some special time with you. For a teenager, it may be more about taking an interest in something they like or making time to enjoy something together.

Building this time in will go a long way towards strengthening your bond with them, reducing their anxiety, and encouraging their development into unique, creative and self-confident individuals, which in my opinion is well worth the few minutes.

Free play

In the end, a playful childhood is the most basic right of childhood.[120]

Childhood serves a real purpose. Being a child is a time of vital preparation for independence in adulthood, with all the joys and challenges this brings – and a childhood wouldn't be a childhood without play.

Free play is exactly what you might expect; typically free of adult supervision, it allows children to explore and experience the world around them. It's unstructured, voluntary and child-initiated, the spontaneous play that comes naturally from children's curiosity, love of discovery and enthusiasm.[121]

'Free play is a fundamental need of all children, which they must have an opportunity to enjoy in order to grow into confident, competent, well-balanced adults. Seen as a testing ground for life, free play provides the experiences children need to acquire the social and emotional skills necessary for healthy psychological development.'[122]

Some children are lucky enough to live in a setting where it's possible for them to play freely with others and their parents allow them to. I would imagine this isn't the case for many other kids, either because of where they live or indeed how our society has changed us.

Unfortunately, over the past half century or so, opportunities for children to play freely with other children without adult supervision have significantly declined. Compared with previous generations, today's kids get fewer opportunities to play freely, because parents understandably fear for their safety, be it on account of fast traffic, bullies or child predators. It's a wonder that we even let our kids out of the front door with all the bad things we hear on the news every day!

Children nowadays spend much of their time in the structured confines of school or engaged in extra-curricular activities. Organised playdates have become the norm instead of spontaneous gatherings of children. Whilst these activities offer a lot of valuable learning and fun for kids, much of their day is spent under the supervision of and directed by adults.

This combination is a double whammy, as it means fewer opportunities for free play, and more activities directed and evaluated by adults, which may be contributing to increased rates of anxiety and depression in children.[123]

> By depriving children of opportunities to play on their
> own, away from direct adult supervision and control,
> we are depriving them of opportunities to learn how to
> take control of their own lives. We may think we are
> protecting them, but in fact we are diminishing their joy,
> diminishing their sense of self-control, preventing them
> from discovering and exploring the endeavours they would
> most love, and increasing the odds that they'll suffer from
> anxiety, depression and other disorders.[124]

Free play is also a natural means of making friends and learning to cooperate with others as equals. When children navigate the rules, there are the endless questions of who will go first, who will be the leader and the follower, and how will we make this work if we both want the same thing? Creative problem-solving like this improves children's brain development, as neural pathways are laid down that they can use again in other situations, such as conflict resolution, in their chosen adult careers.

Because free play is directed and controlled by the players themselves, it provides a vital opportunity for kids to decide what to do and how to do it, to solve their own problems, to follow rules and to keep the game going, all of which help them develop a sense of mastery over their worlds. Just as everyday life brings up lots of emotions for adults, free play does the same for kids. It gives them the chance to learn to regulate positive and negative emotions, which is important for their longer-term emotional health.[125]

Children with anxiety often worry about losing control over their emotions and may even fear their own fear, which makes them less equipped to manage their responses to mildly threat-ening situations. Free play is beneficial because it provides children with the precious opportunity to put themselves into both physically and socially challenging situations, and to learn to control the emotions that arise from these moderately challenging stressors.[126]

Rough-and-tumble play also helps children to manage their feelings better and regain balance. Because there is a constant exchange between our bodies and our brains, changing our physical state through movement has the power to change our emotional state.[127]

Now that you know how beneficial free play is for your child's development and emotional well-being, you may wish to reassess some of the priorities in their current lives.

- Are they getting any time for adult-free play?
- Could a supervised activity be exchanged for a less supervised one?
- Do they get opportunities to resolve their own conflicts before you try to fix things?
- Could you allow them to do one new thing today which you have not let them do up to now?

Perhaps you could begin to identify some small changes in your routine which would allow your child to taste more freedom, excitement and challenge all rolled into one.

Play therapy

> The body heals with play, the mind heals with laughter and
> the spirit heals with joy.
>
> *Proverb*

In my experience, play and creative-therapy approaches have
been helpful with anxious kids of all ages, including teens.
Because anxious children often feel less in control of their
lives and may feel pressurised by other people's judgements,
using play can bring them back to their healthier, carefree
selves.

Play therapy provides a safe opportunity for children to
make sense of their worries and to act out upsetting experiences at their own pace. Using toys instead of words enables
children to transfer their anxieties, fears, fantasies and guilt
onto objects rather than people.[128] By acting out their fears,
children move more closely towards inner resolution, from
which they're better able to cope with challenges and to
become the boss of their worries.

Because 'there is no greater agony than bearing an untold
story inside you',[129] play therapy enables a child to tell their
story in their own way, which helps them to heal.

Play therapy is beneficial for children with any type of
emotional difficulty, including anxiety, particularly those
spanning from pre-school age to adolescence.[130] Younger kids
tend to like sensory forms of play,[131] while older children like
making up stories using symbols and eventually playing these
out themselves.

Anxiety impacts younger children just as significantly as
older children, so it needs to be treated early with appropriate
interventions such as play. Many of you will have heard of a
psychotherapy called cognitive behavioural therapy (CBT).
CBT can be really useful for older children, but less so for

children under eight. Younger children have limited verbal and abstract thinking skills, so this is where play comes in as a great alternative to CBT for infants, toddlers, preschoolers and primary-school kids.[132] Even in middle childhood (ages 8 to 12), play therapy can have a beneficial effect.[133] While play therapy is most often used for children under the age of 13, I have also seen adolescents benefit from using creative approaches.

To give you a real flavour of what play therapy is and how it can help anxious children, I interviewed one of the most playful grown-ups I have ever had the privilege to work with – and play puppets and make yukky slime with! Siobhán Prendiville is a child and adolescent psychotherapist, play therapist, clinical supervisor, author, presenter and trainer. She is the course leader on the Creative Psychotherapy MA at the Children's Therapy Centre in Westmeath, Ireland, and also maintains a private child and adolescent psychotherapy and play-therapy practice. In the case study below, she discusses her play-therapy approach for an anxious little boy she worked with.

It's important to note that, as she says, 'For a child struggling with significant emotional needs, play therapy is best, and most safely and ethically, practised by a mental health professional (e.g. psychotherapist, clinical or counselling psychologist) who can make well-informed decisions based on the child's context.'

• •

A case in point: play therapy and Alex

Malie: How does play therapy help a child with anxiety?

Siobhán: Fear, anxiety, worry are emotions common to us all. My work is not about stopping fear, or blocking it out; rather it's around enabling children to recognise it in themselves and find ways to take control of it, to reduce it, to manage it and to stop it from disturbing their ability to reach their full potential.

I can emphatically say, across the board, that the use of play and creativity in my work is most powerful in enabling children to recognise their fears, counter-condition these fears, develop regulation and coping strategies, and ultimately take control of the fears and worries that initially were controlling them.

Malie: Can you talk me through a scenario when you worked with a child with anxiety?

Siobhán: Eight-year-old Alex came to me for play therapy because his parents were very concerned about his anxious disposition. He was extremely anxious and worried about lots of things, like what to eat and when and where his cat went when he left the house, death, monsters and crime, to name but a few. He had many fears, including the dark and being in the house alone. He suffered from nightmares and found it extremely diffi-cult to fall asleep at night.

Alex was anxious about school; he would often cry when being dropped off and was upset in school regularly. His parents described him as being 'a total worrier' and 'anxious all of the time'. It was clear to me that Alex's anxiety was completely over-whelming and was stopping him from engaging fully in life and in the joys of the world around him.

Malie: When did all this begin for Alex?

Siobhán: In initial sessions with Alex's parents they identified that his anxiety began when he was aged three. They recalled a very scary, traumatic incident that had occurred around this age. However, at the time they had felt that Alex was too young for it to affect him.

Over the years they'd tried various strategies to try to reduce his anxiety. They'd talked to him about his fears and had contin-ually tried to reassure him that he didn't need to be worried. They said these approaches weren't helpful. And so they found me, the 'play lady'.

Malie: I like that, the 'play lady'! So what did you do next to help Alex?

Siobhán: I worked with this family over a five-month period, with a mixture of parent sessions and individual play-therapy sessions for Alex. In parent sessions I supported his parents in empowering them to find suitable ways to help Alex. In the beginning stages, most of this work was about identifying and supporting them with their own anxieties and fears.

Parenting is very challenging, and parenting an anxious child especially so, as it can increase the parents' own anxieties and fears such as: 'What have we done wrong?'; 'Why can't we help him?'; 'Why is he like this?'; 'Will he always be so anxious?'; 'Will his anxiety worsen as he grows older?'

These are very common, and real, parenting worries. It's crucial in my work that we address these worries and help parents to alleviate them, as their ability to be regulated and calm is central to their child's ability to be regulated and calm. Anxiety needs to be met with validation, empathy and calmness.

Malie: I totally agree. It's nearly impossible for a child to regulate themselves if a parent is full up with their own worries. So how did you go about helping Alex's parents?

Siobhán: My focus was on identifying, validating and normalising their worries, and trying to promote their own self-care in between sessions. This was really successful in enabling Alex's parents to better support him. In just a few short weeks we began to see a significant reduction in his parents' own anxiety levels, which had a knock-on effect on Alex's too.

Simple tips I gave the parents in the early stages of therapy included:

- Acknowledge and validate your own feelings as parents. For example: 'I'm worried about Alex, it's scary seeing him so anxious, we're doing what we need to do for him and for us. No feeling lasts forever, we'll get through this.'

- Do what you need to do to stay calm yourself. Find time for yourself: take a bath, go for a walk, listen to your favourite song, have a hot chocolate, dance, etc.
- Acknowledge and validate your child's feelings. Instead of saying, 'You don't need to be worried about going to school, it's really fun in there,' you could say, 'You are worried about going to school today. You do not like being there without me right now. Children and teachers go to school, parents do not. Your teacher knows about your worries and wobbly feelings and she is there to help you with them in school. I'll be keeping you in my heart while you're there, and I'll be at the gate waiting for you at the end of the day.'
- Look out for things that seem to soothe your child when they do experience a big feeling. We want to be able to create a data bank of soothing activities for the child, so the first step is to identify the types of things that generally calm him.

Malie: Great tips there for parents on prioritising their self-care. And I love the idea of a data bank of soothing strategies. How was school going at this point?

Siobhán: School drop-off was still causing distress each morning. To begin to address this I facilitated the telling of a 'structured doll story'[134] with Alex and his parents, where I used small dolls to tell a lively story, playing out the morning routine of dropping Alex off to school, Mum going to work, and Mum coming back to collect Alex at the end of the day.

Malie: How did the doll story help Alex?

Siobhán: He was feeling anxious and insecure about going to school. The story gave him a clear narrative of what was going to happen and focused on the positive aspect of Mum returning to collect him at the end of the school day. It helped Alex to gain a sense of normality and routine about going to school, and therefore it eased his anxiety around it.

Malie: Sounds like a dress-rehearsal for an upcoming performance. Or perhaps the imagining of a fearful situation somehow taking some of the emotional charge out of it?

Siobhán: Exactly like that. And best of all it's a useful technique that parents can use at home as well, following these simple steps:

- The parent creates a story about a real-life situation the child is anxious about, which is occurring in the near future.
- The story involves real-life characters (e.g. Mum, Dad, babysitter, brother, teacher), which are represented by objects (e.g. dolls, figures, pebbles).
- The focus of the story is on the sequence of events (e.g. 'First … then') and on the child's ability to manage the situation with back-up support from trusting adults. An acknowledgement is made that although the child feels anxious, they can gently push through it and feel super-brave afterwards.
- Toys and sound effects can be used to enrich the story and to enhance its dramatic effect. Go to town on it, if you like – the sky's the limit!
- Your child might like to add in a few details of their own to personalise the story.

There is such power in the telling of a story, whether it be before the event to mentally rehearse it, or after an event to process what happened, all at the child's own pace.

Malie: And what were your main goals guiding your work with Alex?

Siobhán: After a few parent sessions, Alex began attending weekly play-therapy sessions with me. These sessions did not focus on Alex's anxiety; instead they focused on Alex. My work is guided by the notion that if given the opportunities to play and speak freely within the context of a trusting child–therapist relationship, children will be able to resolve their own problems and work towards their own solutions.

My goal was to create a safe play space for Alex to attend, to be himself, to play in the ways he wanted to, to form a relationship with me, and through this play and relationship enable him to access the therapeutic powers of play most relevant to him. Alex came, he played, he experienced joy and laughter, and my goodness did he tackle those fears!

Malie: Did you talk directly about his fears with him?

Siobhán: Alex, like other children and teenagers, did not have the words to describe his thoughts and feelings, or his perceptions of his internal and external world. His play brought him to a deeper level than his verbal skills would allow.

Play enables complex thoughts, feelings, ideas and perceptions to be brought into focus. The content of play is informed by the player's personality and current worries.

Alex's play provided him with opportunities to explore his fears through the wonderful dramatic distance that play provides. The scary incident Alex's parents felt he had been too young to be affected by took centre stage in his play. Using role play gave him the chance to try out a new way of being, initially within the safety of the playroom and the play. Through role play, he took his power back. We didn't have to talk about the incident, in order for him to gain healing from it.

Alex grew in confidence before my very eyes in the playroom. He developed a more positive self-concept and become more self-directing, self-accepting and self-reliant. He was better able to cope with anxiety by engaging in soothing activities that helped to calm down his fear response.

Malie: And what kinds of things did you do during the sessions?

Siobhán: I began to identify the play activities that helped to calm Alex down. Blowing bubbles, playing with play dough and dry sand, using stretchy, squidgy and fidget toys, bouncing on a gym ball and listening to music all proved extremely calming for him. Armed with this knowledge I offered suggestions to Alex's parents and teacher around regulating activities to build into his daily routine.

Malie: And how did this work translate back to his home environment?

Siobhán: Once I got to know Alex, further work with his parents shifted to including more daily play-based routines at home. Individual therapy sessions continued during this time as Alex integrated all the shifts and changes he had made through this amazing therapy journey in my special playroom. These included:

- The use of daily positive affirmations:
    'I am strong'
    'I am calm'
    'I am confident'
    'I can breathe deeply'
    'I believe in me'
    'I can do this'
    'I am a special star, I shine bright'
    'I have many gifts and talents'
    'I am relaxed and in control of my feelings'
    'I can ask for help when I need it'
    'Today is going to be a great day'

- Using calming strategies: blowing bubbles, playing with play dough, squidgy toys, fidget spinners and sand; offering back rubs and hand massages, etc.
- Using a worry puppet called Walter, who was accompanied by a box filled with notes on a selection of calming strategies: blow bubbles, bounce on a ball, listen to music, etc. The box also included little worry cards, on which Alex could draw or write any worry he had. Alex and his parents

began to use this regularly, meaning that Alex was now
sharing his worries with Walter, and of course his parents,
and being given a technique that helped to ease his anxiety.

- Being read therapeutic stories at bedtime to help Alex
  explore his emotions and practise visualisations.
- Play! Alex's parents began spending more time playing with
  Alex, allowing him to take the lead in the play.

Malie: How did it all turn out in the end?

Siobhán: After 12 individual sessions, Alex's parents described
having their 'boy back'. They said he was 'lighter', 'happier' and
'far less anxious'.

School drop-off was no longer an issue. Alex was now happy
going to school and teacher reports indicated that he had started
partaking in many everyday class activities, which he had not
done before.

The shifts and changes I'd seen in Alex and his play in the
therapy room were transferring over into his real world. Playing
with anxiety had truly empowered Alex – and his parents. The
confident, self-assured, happy young boy showed me just how
much the magically therapeutic powers of play had been hard
at work!

Not every child needs to see a play therapist, although many
would benefit. The above case study provides you with ideas
that you can hopefully bring home to regulate your child
during anxious moments, to increase their control and to
engage their problem-solving skills, all while deepening your
connection and having fun. Not a bad day's work!

Play techniques for parents

Because children with anxiety spend much of their time 'on guard' – on the lookout for danger, parents using play techniques in this way can help to bring some much-needed light and laughter into the panic station zone. This is especially helpful if you're also prone to anxiety as a parent.

Playing with anxiety in this way shows your child that you're not overwhelmed by their fears, that you're game for a bit of fun, and that you're both telling the annoying worries to take a hike by not feeding them any more.

• •

A case in point: silly-fying the fear

Eight-year-old Tommy had been having recurring nightmares about monsters, which scared the life out of him. After a few sessions, I asked him to draw the monsters as a way of making them less scary and creating some distance from them.

Tommy was unsure about this at first. I totally understood his uncertainty as we were addressing one of his fears, so I made sure to give him full control over his creation and the pace at which he wanted to drive the exercise.

'Many kids I've seen have found it helpful to draw something they're afraid of,' I told him, 'because it often seems less scary in the light of day, when everything feels a bit safer. How about we start by drawing the least scary dream for today, and see how we get on? We can add in as much or as little detail as you like, and you can tell me when you'd like to move on.'

Tommy bravely agreed. He sketched the sequence of the previous night's dream. It was all about a monster with big orange eyes and very long limbs chasing after him and his sister.

I wondered whether the monster had a name. Tommy said he was called Mr Googly.

Tommy used a black marker pen to draw the scene and used a black pastel to shade the background. I asked him to tell me the story frame by frame, slowly, and to refer to the monster as Mr Googly.

'Me and my sister were running, running, running, trying to get away from Mr Googly. He was roaring at us to come back. We built a tall wall to stop him, but he just climbed over it so easily! We were running as fast as we could down a steep slope, not knowing where we'd end up. We found a ladder in the middle of nowhere and decided to climb it. We had no other way to escape. We kept climbing up and up like Jack and his beanstalk. Mr Googly was still chasing after us, climbing two steps at a time. When we got up to the roof, he grabbed my sister and I had to pull her back with all of my strength. Then we both jumped off the roof towards the water below. I woke up before I landed in the water.'

I asked Tommy was there anything he could do to make the monster look silly or a bit less scary? He thought about it and said, 'I don't know.' I suggested a big red hat and a nappy. Tommy laughed and drew these on. I wondered, could he imagine Mr Googly with hiccups or talking baby talk? Tommy said he could, but didn't know if he could do that in the dream.

When asked what might have happened if he hadn't woken up, Tommy said that he and his sister would have swum away, but the monster would probably have caught up with them. I wondered if maybe the monster's lanky arms and long legs might tangle him up and stop him from swimming? Tommy said maybe they would.

I wondered, could anything slow Mr Googly down, like wearing giant roller skates? Tommy said that was a silly idea and that Mr Googly was just too fast in his dream.

At this point, Tommy asked to move on to something else, which we did. It was clear that he had gone as far as he could, so I didn't push it. However, something really interesting happened later in the session.

Tommy soaked a sponge with water and said, 'I know a way to make my dream less scary.' He carried the wet sponge to the table and squeezed it over his picture. The ink began to run and he rubbed out Mr Googly with the sponge, slowly at first, then much faster. He wet the sponge a few more times, then rolled up the wet paper into a big soggy ball and flung it right in the bin.

When Tommy came back the following week, he said Mr Googly had gone away. We still had other fears and dream monsters to silly-fy, but at least Tommy had found a way to conquer one of them in his own way.

 For another fun approach to playing with anxiety, flip ahead to 'Giving your worry a name' in the Appendices on page 241.

Cognitive behavioural therapy and anxiety

Our thinking creates our feelings and behaviour, and when our minds are calm we have access to natural wisdom and healthy feelings.[135]

Treatment of anxiety and cognitive behavioural therapy (CBT) go hand in hand. In this day and age, when young people often feel overwhelmed by their negative thoughts, CBT offers something very tangible to calm their minds so they can regain access to their natural wisdom. CBT is a talking therapy that helps children over the age of eight, teens and adults manage their problems through changing the way they think and the way they behave by seeking more helpful alternatives. It's based on the assumption that feelings and behaviours are largely a product of our thinking, and that negative thoughts, feelings and behaviours trap us in a vicious cycle. CBT aims to help crack this cycle by breaking down overwhelming problems into smaller parts, and by offering practical tools to change negative thinking and behaviour patterns to improve the way we feel in our minds and in our bodies.

In a nutshell, CBT focuses on the relationship between:

- what I think
- how I feel
- what I do
- how my body feels

CBT works well with anxiety because it engages the reasoning part of the brain to calm the body down, to challenge negative thoughts and to reduce the tendency to avoid fears. It's important to note that if a child is in a deep panic they'll need anchoring and feeling felt techniques before moving on to challenging their thoughts or facing their fears.

Most parents I see wonder what may have caused their child's anxiety and if they might have contributed to it in any way. Whilst genes and temperament predispose a child to becoming anxious, and the environment also plays an important role, *no single factor* causes a child's anxiety. Typically there are a number of factors at play.

Although it can be helpful to understand *why* your child is anxious, it's not essential.[136] What is more important in making anxiety better is to understand what is *maintaining* a child's anxiety or keeping it going. This is where CBT comes into its own, as it looks at the impact of negative thoughts and behaviours on a child's feelings in their mind and body. CBT also offers a very clear way out of this vicious cycle by teaching children and parents skills to find positive ways of coping with anxiety.

Many anxious children make negative predictions about how a situation will turn out, which can lead to them experiencing uncomfortable bodily symptoms and avoiding the situation. The problem with avoidance is that the child never gets a chance to test out their predictions! They assume that because they feel afraid, they *must* be in danger, even if they're not. Avoidance makes them feel worse, so it's a vicious cycle that keeps going around and around.

To work out your child's vicious cycle, have a look back at the section entitled 'Thinking about anxiety as a cycle' on page 117, and discuss it with your child. Pick a situation that makes your child anxious and ask them the following questions:

- 'What are the anxious thoughts that go through your mind?'
- 'What do you feel in your body? How do you react?'
- 'What do you do or avoid doing? How does this make you feel?'

CBT in action for children and teenagers with anxiety
To give you a real flavour of how CBT can help anxious children and teenagers, I interviewed Pamela Carroll Mannion, an amazing psychotherapist I had the pleasure of working alongside in a Child and Adolescent Mental Health Service (CAMHS) many years ago.[137]

• •

A case in point: CBT and Tom

Malie: What would you say is the youngest age a child can engage in and benefit from CBT?

Pamela: To be able to engage in CBT, a child must have a certain level of understanding so that they can think about their thoughts, as in identify, challenge and find alternative, more healthy thoughts. They must also be able to 'think outside the box' and view situations from different perspectives. With this in mind, children from the age of eight years are usually suitable to engage in CBT, but this can vary from individual to individual and include factors like a young person's social and family context, and their temperament.

Malie: Would you use the same techniques with children as you would with adults?

Pamela: CBT needs to be adapted when working with a younger age group. Games might be used to help engage young people or you might reward them when they have participated well in a session. A sense of fun during sessions can really help to loosen things up, reduce discomfort in problems being explored and help to build the all-important client–therapist relationship.

Malie: Do you include parents in the CBT treatment?

Pamela: Absolutely, as they're the ones best placed to support their children between sessions. Usually I ask that a parent join at the beginning of a session to help give feedback about how the previous week has been, as well as at the end of the session for general feedback about the session and how they can help their child use the skills that week. Schools can also be included if needed.

Malie: What does CBT therapy look like in practice?

Pamela: CBT prides itself on:

- Collaboration: the young person and therapist work together to achieve goals for therapy, and everything is done in an open way so that the family feels empowered to help themselves.
- Time-limited: sessions are weekly, lasting an hour, and the therapy usually goes on for between 16 and 20 sessions in total, sometimes less. Changes can often be seen in the young person after six sessions.
- 'Here and now' focus: CBT does not focus on the past. Instead, it looks to the present and to the future, focusing on new and more proactive ways of managing life.

- Skills-based approach: CBT teaches clients alternative ways of thinking and behaving so that they'll feel better. It's vital to the success of therapy that these skills be practised regularly during the sessions but also outside of them with the encouragement of parents.
- Self-discovery and experimentation: the young person learns to question their thoughts and patterns of behaviour through a process of experimentation, which helps them to discover new ways of thinking and behaving.

Malie: Can you talk me through a scenario when you worked with a child with anxiety?

Pamela: Tom was 12 years old, lived with his parents and two younger siblings, and was in his final class in a small primary school. He was complaining of 'pains in his tummy and head, getting very upset at times, having trouble breathing and experiencing heart palpitations'. Although Tom was academically bright, his parents reported that he was starting to fall behind in his schoolwork and didn't want to sleep on his own at night. Tom attended with me for 12 CBT sessions in total.

Malie: Did Tom share with you what was going on with him and causing him such distress?

Pamela: Yes, he was really open and spoke about his fears of going to secondary school, not being able to cope with all his new subjects and the pressure of exams, getting lost in such a big school and looking stupid in front of his peers. His fear of the unknown led to him predicting that the worst would happen. Secondary school was looking scarier the closer it came. He was also sad to be leaving his primary school, where he felt safe and knew everyone.

Despite much reassurance from his parents that he would be OK, Tom wasn't so sure. His mother also had a history of being anxious; unfortunately, this resulted in Tom worrying excessively about his mother worrying about him!

Malie: That sounds like a vicious circle, and is not uncommon in my experience. How did Tom feel about his parents bringing him to you for help?

Pamela: Tom was really motivated to change. He was so fed up feeling really worried and sad that he had even Googled CBT before coming in. He was optimistic that the sessions would help, and his parents were very much on board, as were his school, who said they were happy to help.

Malie: Everyone being on board is a really positive start. What did you do to assess Tom?

Pamela: Once I got a good picture from Tom and his parents of his struggles and background history, he filled out some questionnaires measuring the severity of his anxiety and its impact on his daily life. This was done again at the end of sessions to measure progress made. Next, I spoke to him and to his parents, and we explored how CBT might help him to cope better with his anxiety.

Malie: How did Tom and his parents react to you saying that your goal was for him to cope better with anxiety rather than get rid of it, as many clients would understandably wish for?

Pamela: As with many clients, I needed to set realistic expectations for the treatment. Because Tom had a history of being anxious from quite a young age, it was more realistic for us to work on empowering Tom with an 'anxiety toolkit' instead of an 'anxiety destroyer', so to speak. Once Tom had come up with treatment goals to work on, we focused on helping him to understand what was happening to him: 'Worry is normal; it protects us from danger. But sometimes it gets a little out of control and we need to take that control back again.' Tom began recognising that his heart palpitations, headaches and difficulties breathing were caused by worry. His worrying thoughts about secondary school were caused by anxiety and while reassurance helped for a little while, they soon came back, especially at night time.

Although we can never make anxiety go away completely, there are ways of managing it better. One of these was to ask Tom what his anxiety looked like. Tom drew a picture of a large scary creature, with sharp teeth, a long tail, big bloodshot eyes, a pointy nose and huge smelly feet. From then on he was going to visualise this creature playing tricks on him, sending him these awful thoughts and physical symptoms, and causing him so much worry. Tom and I explored ways he could boss back the creature to regain control of his anxiety.

Amazingly this technique was also helpful to his mother. Tom enjoyed becoming the anxiety expert and even encouraged his mother to boss back her anxiety too!

Malie: That must have felt amazing for Tom to be able to help himself and his mum too. What happened next?

Pamela: We then focused on encouraging Tom to put his anxiety into words in a Thought Diary. It's not an event itself that causes feelings of anxiety; rather it's a person's *response* to the event – their mindset – that plays a crucial role. Hence it was important to explore Tom's thoughts in response to situations. What were his negative automatic thoughts (NATs) when he noticed himself feeling worried or when his heart was racing?

Malie: What exactly are negative automatic thoughts?

Pamela: Negative automatic thoughts are the running commentary going on in our heads. Because we allow NATs to play in our minds continuously, they become habitual, which makes us more likely to believe them and not look for evidence to the contrary. When we accept these negative thoughts as true, it has a knock-on effect on how we feel and on what we do. For this reason it's really important to remember that thoughts are opinions and not facts, and, like all opinions, they may not be true.

Tom's unhelpful thoughts included:

- 'I won't be able to do it.'
- 'What if I fail my exams?'
- 'What if people won't like me?'
- 'Everyone else can do it.'
- 'They're all laughing at me.'

Malie: So what did you do with Tom's list of thoughts?

Pamela: We explored Tom's thoughts and the possibility that he might be making mistakes in his thinking. These 'thinking traps'[138] are the ways our mind convinces us of one thing when in reality it might be completely untrue. In Tom's situation, it became clear that the nature of his NATs resulted in him experiencing unpleasant feelings like anxiety, physical sensations like a sore tummy, changes in his behaviour like not wanting to sleep on his own, and falling behind on schoolwork.

Malie: All of which were maintaining his cycle of anxiety.

Pamela: That's it exactly! I spoke to Tom about the different types of thinking traps and those most relevant to him. I encouraged him to put his negative thoughts on trial, with questions like:

- 'Is that an opinion or a fact? How so?'
- 'Am I jumping to conclusions/mind reading/seeing in black and white? How so?'
- 'What evidence do I have?'
- 'Are there any alternative explanations?'

Later, I asked Tom to take a more realistic and balanced perspective, which looked something like:

- 'I won't be able to do it' *became* 'It'll take time to adjust, but I'm smart and settle pretty well into new things.'
- 'What if people don't like me?' *became* 'I'm popular in school and on the football team, so there's no reason why it won't be the same in my new school.'

- 'Everyone else can do it' *became* 'I can too. I just need to take it one day at a time. My teachers say I'm ready to move on.'
- 'They're all laughing at me' *became* 'I have no evidence that anyone is laughing at me. That's just my anxiety playing tricks on me.'

With the help of his parents, Tom began noticing that questioning his worried thoughts led to him finding more balanced alternative thoughts instead, which improved his mood and his levels of anxiety.

Malie: That's a great improvement! And did you suggest a specific time each day for Tom to challenge his thoughts?

Pamela: We agreed to have a 'worry time' of ten minutes each night before bedtime when Tom talked to one or both parents about his worries, challenged them and distracted himself with other happier thoughts, allowing him to settle to sleep more easily. If Tom had negative thoughts during the day, he had a choice of bossing back his anxiety then using his Thought Diary, or he could save his worries for 'worry time'.

'Worry time' worked really well for Tom before bed, allowing him to empty his head of worries and soon he was sleeping by himself again. This also allowed for a better night's sleep, with Tom feeling less tired, and more able to concentrate and keep up with his schoolwork. It was also helping his mood, as he appeared happier and more relaxed. His parents reported that the witty, funny character that he used to be had started to return!

By the end of eight sessions, Tom was feeling much better in himself as he had achieved his therapy goals. However, his anxiety began to rise when the countdown to the first school day began, especially worries about taking the school bus, as he had always been dropped to the school gate by his parents (i.e. 'What if I miss the bus?; What if I don't get a seat?').

Malie: So many anxious kids are prone to 'What if' thinking, which is often resistant to logic. How did you help him?

Pamela: The best way was to focus on the opposite of 'What if' which is 'What is', and the reality of the here-and-now moment. Encouraging children to check in with how their bodies feel as they ask 'What if' questions anchors them into the present. Helping them to use practised ways to calm themselves down, like relaxation techniques, works well too.

Now that we had looked at Tom's thoughts and feelings on the CBT triangle (see page 118), the next step was to focus on his behaviour by designing a fear ladder to test out his negative predictions about taking the school bus.

Learning any scary new behaviour needs to be broken down into tiny steps, which are mastered one by one. This type of gradual exposure is particularly helpful if a child has a phobia or avoids certain situations.

Malie: What was the outcome of Tom's fear ladder?

Pamela: It worked really well as Tom was very motivated to reach his goal and had good support from his parents and friend. Once he had gotten on the bus himself and managed a few journeys, he became more confident. He realised there were plenty of other new kids and even began to enjoy the fun and freedom of it! We all praised Tom on his courage in having bossed back his negative thoughts and his fear. As for his 'What if' thoughts, I encouraged him to assertively say back to himself 'IF it happens, THEN I'll deal with it'.

Malie: That is so empowering. How much longer did you work with Tom?

Pamela: By the mid-term break Tom had settled well into his new school and he and his parents were happy for us to end sessions. Tom and his family were such a pleasure to work with, their motivation to change and commitment to coming to sessions certainly lent to the success of the therapy.

Malie: Thanks so much for that, Pamela. It was a great taster of what parents can expect from CBT sessions with children. Would you have any special tips for them?

Pamela: If you notice your child is anxious, here are a few suggestions:

- Before talking to your child about their anxiety, ensure that you yourself are relaxed, have plenty of time and won't be interrupted.
- Describe a situation in which you noticed them being anxious or worried about something. Gently ask them, 'Is everything OK?'
- *No worry is a silly worry!* If it's causing your child to be distressed, then it's a big deal to them.
- Ask them to draw what anxiety looks like (e.g. a 'worry monster'), so they can distance themselves from it and see it as playing tricks with them.
- Reassure them that anxiety is normal. Give them an example of a time when you felt anxious and how you managed it, and tell them you're both going to work together to boss back their worries. If you feel their anxiety is too big to handle yourselves, get some professional help.
- Deep-breathing techniques can help calm things down and are nice to practise together.
- If your child is good at talking about their thoughts, then using a 'worry box' or having 'worry time' is a constructive way for them to express their worries.
- If your child is getting very upset by their worries or is acting out then having a 'calm box' and 'calm space' can be helpful. A 'calm box' includes things to soothe all the child's senses. Pick items with special meaning to your child: comfort blanket, stuffed animal, favourite book or music, stress ball, etc. A 'calm space' is a nurturing place to go to relax, either in the house or outside in nature, as long as it allows your child some quiet time. This can also be a space for a parent to join if invited.

- Praise, praise and lots of it ... no matter how small the achievement.
- A *final* tip for parents is the need for self-care, as it's essential to have the emotional batteries charged to cope with the challenges that each day brings.

Mindfulness meets kindfulness

A few years ago when people shared their positive experiences with mindfulness, I couldn't help but think what exactly does 'mindfulness' mean and why are people raving about it? Because I put myself under pressure with most things (here I am writing on a Friday night!), I felt a bit like the only one who hadn't got aboard the mindfulness bandwagon and was rather cynical about it all.

This was a mistake. And I'll tell you why. But first let me get my old prejudices out of the way. Mindfulness can be given a bad rap nowadays as people see it as something they must 'get right' like everything else in their lives, or as a fad that will pass as easily as it came. The truth is that all of us can be mindful in little ways every day, and with practice, mindfulness can really bolster our emotional well-being:

> You don't need to be broken or be hippy or even spiritual to practise mindfulness ... We need to break the distrust and illusion that mindfulness is some type of quick fix or mumbo jumbo that requires you to wear tie dye or burn incense. The truth is our brains are not geared for the fast-paced, technology-driven twenty-first century, where everything needs to happen in an instant. Neuroscience is telling us that. It's also telling us that with practice, it's possible to make changes in the brain to increase our overall sense of well-being and happiness.[139]

As concerns mount about the societal pressures children face, ways of tackling stress and anxiety and building resilience are coming into focus. In recent years, mindfulness has come to the fore as a valuable tool in helping people of all ages cope with these pressures.

> We all have to accept and move with societal changes, but we also need to ensure that we don't let the price of changing times be paid by our children. We need to implement coping strategies and programmes to make sure children have a chance to still grow up into confident, happy, kind, loving and creative adults, despite the challenges they face. Mindfulness can play a substantial role in arming our children with such strategies.[140]

In addition to self-kindness and common humanity, one of the three central qualities of self-compassion is mindfulness. All three combine and mutually interact to create a self-compassionate state of mind.

> Regular mindfulness practice brings an increased awareness of what influences us, such as our thoughts, emotions, environment and physical sensations. This moment-by-moment awareness allows us to choose what's helpful for us to focus on, experience or do, rather than simply live our lives on automatic pilot.[141]

Research indicates that mindfulness helps children to manage their negative feelings like anxiety, sadness and anger, and improves their self-worth and overall well-being.[142] When children learn to be more 'present' in the moment, they can pay better attention and make wiser decisions because they have engaged the reasoning part of their brain.

What tends to happen when children are anxious is that their minds get busier and their bodies get tenser. This can turn into a vicious circle, with one feeding off the other. Mindfulness helps to break this pattern through the use of attention. By moving our attention from our thoughts to how our bodies feel, we can learn to deliberately relax our bodies so that our mind now gets a different message – a much calmer one.

In an effort to make mindfulness more accessible, the Wheel of Awareness meditation was developed as an exercise that can be used for older children and adults to help them develop their focus of attention.[143]

Our mind can be pictured as a bicycle wheel, with a hub at the centre and spokes radiating towards the outer rim. The rim represents anything we can pay attention to or become aware of: our thoughts and feelings, our dreams and desires, our memories, our perceptions of the outside world and our bodily sensations. The hub is the inner mind, from which we become aware of all that's happening around us and within us. Almost like the control tower!

Children sometimes need a picture to help them understand difficult concepts, so the Wheel of Awareness in the Appendices (see page 260) can show them that their different thoughts and feelings are simply different points on their wheel and particular aspects of themselves that they don't need to give so much attention to.[144]

Mindfulness in practice

One person who demystified the benefits of mindfulness for me is children's therapist and mindfulness teacher Louise Shanagher.[145]

She is also author of the *Mindfully Me* book series for children,[146] and after road-testing the storybooks on my girls – who gave a big thumbs-up – I really wanted to interview Louise and to share it with you.

• •

A case in point

Malie: Louise, for those who aren't familiar with it, what is mindfulness?

Louise: Mindfulness is the practice of paying attention to the present moment, on purpose and without judgement. It's a practical and effective self-care tool that helps children to relax, clear their minds and manage difficult situations, thoughts and feelings. Mindfulness helps children to connect with themselves, increasing confidence, self-awareness and well-being. One of the best things about it is that it's free, can be done almost anywhere and, once learned, can become an invaluable tool for life.

Malie: How did you get into the whole area of mindfulness?

Louise: Working in adult and teenage psychotherapy, it really hit home how big an issue depression and anxiety had become. I felt that both of these needed to be addressed in children at an earlier stage. I was amazed and frustrated that children were not routinely taught how to manage their emotions. It seemed really obvious, and society would reap so many rewards if we invested more in this area for children from early on. The benefits would be far-reaching.

Children aren't taught how to be emotionally well. They are taught how to achieve and how to have a career. They aren't often exposed to conversations about how we relate to ourselves and within our relationships, how we interact with our environment, and how our brains and emotions work.

I started with the children's creative meditation classes. I want to help in normalising our inner world, our thoughts and feelings, our struggles, and teaching children effective tools to manage issues in their life. In teaching mindfulness to children I've found that many seem to have a very harsh inner critic, like an inner bully. What I try to do is encourage them to have kindness and compassion towards themselves.

Malie: What is the relationship between mindfulness and self-compassion?

Louise: As my own mindfulness practice developed, I began to notice the frequency of my self-critical thoughts and how I tended to be very hard on myself. Mindfulness alone, without engaging the emotions, can lead to a sort of emotional alienation. There can be a lack of warmth with just doing mindfulness. Having a kind attitude towards yourself is just as important as paying mindful attention. The two need to go hand in hand.

After experiencing the benefits of mindfulness and self-compassion for myself and wishing I had come across these practices earlier in life, I began my current work teaching children and families how to develop these skills.

Malie: How can parents help their children with mindfulness and self-compassion?

Louise: For parents, the most important place to start is always with their own relationship with themselves. We are teaching children what we are, not necessarily what we say. If we want our children to be mindful, to love and accept themselves, then we need to model this for them first. Self-compassion is very much a practice and takes time to develop. It's not about being perfect, but is instead a continual commitment to a friendship with ourselves.

It's also very important to bring a sense of kindness and friendship to our attention. So many parents can be self-critical, comparing themselves with other parents and feeling they're just not good enough. Instead, try developing a kind, non-judgemental relationship with yourself.

I think one of the best questions to ask ourselves is: am I being a good friend to myself in this moment?

And if not, ask yourself:

• How can I be a better friend to myself?
• How can I care for myself differently?

- How can I speak to myself differently?
- How can I be kinder to myself?

Malie: Any other suggestions for parents?

Louise: Children often have big feelings, and one of the most beneficial things parents can do is to normalise their child's feelings. I would encourage families to spend time openly discussing feelings together. Children can often believe it's bad or wrong to experience certain feelings.

Parents can talk to children about the feelings they felt when they were younger and the ones they still feel as adults. It can be a nice idea to spend time at the end of the day where each family member talks about the feelings they experienced today and what prompted them. Always reassure your child that there are no bad or wrong feelings. Although some feelings can be uncomfortable, we can learn how to manage those feelings and ask for help.

Malie: In your experience, at what age can children begin to learn the skills of mindfulness?

Louise: Mindfulness is a skill that we can teach children from three years of age, and is a great tool that they can use to cope with difficult thoughts, emotions and situations.

As a start, I'd encourage parents to set aside one minute each day for the family to practise mindful breathing together. Good times to practise are either in the morning – or in the evening as a wind down before bed. Start off with five breaths and increase to ten breaths; and then to 30 seconds and 60 seconds. As your child gets used to practising, you can increase the time. Here's how:

Ask your child to put their hand on their belly, and to feel it move in and out as they breathe. Another way is to invite your child to put their fingers under their nose and focus on the feeling of cold air on their fingers as they breathe in and warm air as they breathe out. Your child could also put a small soft toy (their breathing buddy) on their tummy, and watch or feel the toy move up and down with their breathing.

Remind your child that now is a time to relax their mind and to notice what their breathing feels like. Explain that when they breathe this way it helps them to pay attention to what is happening in the here and now. It means not thinking about something that has happened already or something that might happen in the future.

Explain to your child that their thoughts and feelings are just like clouds in the sky, and that they're always changing and moving, never staying the same. Assure your child that if their mind wanders to another thought, let the thought drift away like a cloud and invite them to gently bring their focus back to their breathing.

Remind your child that, like the blue sky behind the clouds, their breath is always there. You can assure them that no matter what is happening in their lives and however they're feeling, that they can always connect with their breath like this. Remember – 'It's always there.'[147]

You can encourage your child to practise a few mindful breaths anytime they feel their mind is busy or when they would like to feel more calm. The great thing about mindful breathing is that they can practise it at their desk in school, before a match, or in the schoolyard – and nobody else needs to know. For children who are prone to anxiety, it's a good idea to build this in when they're calm so they have it in their toolbox when feeling worried. As an add-on, if your child is feeling worried ask them to locate the emotion in their body, to put their hand gently over this place and to practise talking to themselves in the same way they would talk to a good friend.

Malie: I love it, it's like their own secret calming potion they can use whenever they like! Mindful breathing could be really helpful as a daily practice for children and parents who often feel over-whelmed by the busyness of their daily lives and schedules.

Louise: Absolutely. I think it can be very helpful for parents to take a step back and look at what's really important for your children from a broader perspective. Ask yourself: *'What is it I really want for my child?'* Often the answer comes down to us wanting happiness and well-being for our children more than anything else. A different question we can then ask is: *'How can I best support my child's happiness and well-being today and in the coming days and weeks?'*

....

Cultivating kindfulness in children

Kindness + self-compassion + mindfulness = kindfulness

When I brewed up the subtitle to this book – A compassionate approach to parenting your anxious child – I was thinking about parents nurturing compassion in themselves and in their children. Increasingly, researchers are finding that the key to a happy and fulfilled life is resilience. Well, guess what? The key to resilience is kindfulness.

Self-compassion is about nurturing our relationship with ourselves and learning to be our own good friend. When kids who are struggling practise self-compassion, powerful things can happen: they experience a boost in their brain's feel-good chemicals, which lowers stress, and relieves anxiety and low mood; and their sense of self-worth, resilience and ability to cope with challenges improves.

Showing kindness towards others is something that also deeply resonates with me. I'm an emotional wreck every time I watch programmes like *The Secret Millionaire* or anything that shows the beauty of human kindness. It makes me feel all warm and fuzzy inside. It shows me that the world can be a really good place:

Kindness can jumpstart a cascade of positive social
consequences. Helping others leads people to like you,
appreciate you, to offer gratitude. It also may lead people
to reciprocate in your times of need. Helping others can
satisfy a basic human need for connecting with others,
winning you smiles, thankfulness and valued friendship.

Sonja Lyubomirsky

This is what common humanity is all about. Kindness is literally contagious.

A local Volunteer Galway wellness initiative I was most
happy to promote emanated from a Volunteer Ireland study[148]
that found a positive link between helping others and overall
feelings of well-being for the volunteer. Benefits included feeling useful, purposeful and valued; feeling connected to the
community and a sense of belonging; and feeling a sense of
perspective on life and appreciation for life's blessings.

In adults, performing regular acts of kindness (i.e. six times
a week for four weeks) was linked with a relaxed mood, an
increase in relationship satisfaction and a reduction in anxiety.[149] The most likely explanation is that helping others helps
an anxious person to take a break from the stressors in their
own lives and teaches them coping skills for handling future
stressful situations. For those with emotional challenges who
may otherwise be more used to seeking support, the feeling of
making a difference to someone else's life can be life-changing.

It's possible to help a child build their compassion 'muscles'
and respond to others with care. Can you imagine a school
where kindfulness training was adopted into the curriculum?
I'm quite certain we would see a rise in emotional resilience
and a decrease in bullying and mental health issues.

Modelling self-compassion relates to our ability to manage
our own feelings as parents. Difficulties don't arise from the
feelings themselves, but rather from not being able to express

them in a healthy way. By loving ourselves through mistakes and negative experiences, we give our children a solid foundation for the future:

> [Children need a] foundation for being kind and gentle with themselves and processing their thoughts and feelings without judgement. These are important skills for being a healthy adult and building healthy relationships.[150]

Here are a few suggestions for helping children to incorporate kindfulness into their lives:

Inner kindness voice

We all speak to ourselves unkindly sometimes, which has huge power over how we feel and how we make sense of our experiences. Just like adults, children can be their own worst critics and judge themselves very harshly, which can start from an early age. They may be comparing themselves to others and feel they don't quite measure up in some way.

Repetitive critical self-talk can lead to low self-worth and increased anxiety. Explain to your children that an inner bully is something we *all* experience. We can help children to combat their critical self-talk by cultivating self-compassion or kindfulness.

A great book that teaches helpful self-kindness tools in a very simple and child-friendly way is Fiona Forman's *Self-Kindness for Kids: Whizzo-Voice to the Rescue!*[151] In the book, children are encouraged to become aware of their inner bully voice and are introduced to their kinder inner voice, who helps to turn the inner bully voice down.

Providing children with tangible tools for encouraging their compassionate voice to calm their inner bully is invaluable. In her work with schools, Fiona encourages students to draw Kind Mind posters of kind things they can say to themselves:

'I'm good enough', 'I don't need to be perfect', 'Focus on the positive things', 'I'm not alone' and 'I don't need to compare myself to anyone.' Pure wisdom there.

Mantras

Another way of encouraging children to develop a kinder inner voice and of building their ability to cope in the face of daily stresses is through the use of mantras. Mantras are particularly good for children with anxiety as they encourage them to deliberately generate positive thoughts that not only have the power to calm their anxious feelings but can also help them to stop avoiding challenges.

What I love about mantras is that they're positive and children remember them easily. When I told my youngest about my book title, we made up this thing where I say 'Love in', she gives me a loud smooch, and she says 'Love out', cue another smooch! My eldest daughter had a different take on it: 'Mummy, if you put love into your heart, then your child can put all their love out into the world.' My heart just melted … kindfulness, there it was.

A good place to start is for parents to come up with a mantra of their own. So while one of mine is *'Love in, love out'*, yours could be something that is really meaningful to your experience or that makes you smile. Examples include *'Breathe'*, *'It's OK'*, *'This too shall pass'*, *'It is what it is'*, *'Try a hug'*, *'Namaste'* – whatever floats your boat!

Ideas for mantras come from all sorts of places, like the lyrics of a song or a really good quote that makes you feel whole and loved. Once you have chosen yours, maybe you could share it with your child and invite them to come up with a few good ones of their own to help calm their anxious moments. Here are a few more:

'Be the pond'[152]

One of my favourite mantras for all children, especially children with anxiety, was developed by a teacher to explain a busy mind. This exercise encourages children to take a step back from their feelings and to watch them as if they're fish swimming by in a pond, without being ruled by them. Talk to your child about what it means to be the pond and highlight their ability to pay attention to what they choose to pay attention to. When we forget that we're the pond, and think that that we're the anxious fish, then the anxious fish makes us really scared and avoid things. But being the pond, we can focus on things that make us feel brave and able for the world.

Because children have vast imaginations, using metaphors like this is great for teaching them to mindfully observe their feelings and thoughts without engaging or judging them. When they feel anxious or sad, which they will because they're human, they can notice the feeling and realise that it will eventually swim away and a different one will soon swim along.

'Let it go'

Some of us are totally sick of the song 'Let It Go' from the Disney film *Frozen* by now (my daughters flogged it to death!), but these three words can be a powerful mantra for children and parents alike, as the phrase recognises that there are many things we can't control. 'Let it go' is less about suppressing or denying our emotions, it's more about putting our minds, especially our children's developing reasoning brains, back in control of the emotion centres in the brain so we can figure out what to do next.

'I am thankful'

Many of us spend a lot of time chasing what we don't have rather than celebrating what we do have. It's like we're on this endless treadmill searching for a destination that we'll never reach. It's a trap and we can all get caught up on this silly journey sometimes. So how can we get off the treadmill?[153]

A great way to counterbalance our brain's default tendency to find negativity is to practise gratitude (*'I'm thankful'*). It all makes sense when you think that for every negative thought, we need five positives to even things out. That's a lot of gratitude.

As a family or when you're alone with your child, share one thing you're grateful for each day. Today my youngest said 'Chocolate', which, to be fair, I'm grateful for too! Her second offering was 'My family', a warm reminder for many of us that we're surrounded by abundance, by the special people we love who love us back, by what brings us real joy and laughter in life, and that we have a home to live in.

Affirmation cards

Affirmations are statements that help us to overcome our inner bully thoughts and help us to visualise and create positive changes in our lives.

Making affirmation cards with your child is a good way of encouraging them to speak more kindly to themselves.[154] Create affirmations to suit the needs of your own child. Affirmations such as *'I'm just right'*, *'I'm loved'* or *'I'm safe'* will work well for most children. For children with worries or fears, affirmations acknowledging their feelings and emphasising their sense of safety can work really well. You can encourage your child to say things to themselves like:

- 'I'm feeling scared now, and I don't like how it feels, but I know that it's OK to have this feeling.'
- 'Everyone feels scared sometimes. There are lots of other children who are feeling just like me.'

- 'Even though I feel scared, I know that I'm OK, I'm safe and I'm loved. I know I can always ask for help when I have this feeling.'

Once you've picked a few, get some small pieces of card and write an affirmation on each one. Be as creative as you like! Next, ask your child to draw a picture or stick images on it.

As children repeat their affirmations, it can also be really helpful to encourage them to use self-soothing touch, by giving themselves a little hug or putting their hand on their heart.

You can repeat positive affirmations with your child at any time of the day or when they're feeling particularly anxious about something. You could pop some affirmation cards in their bag that they could use during the day as an anchor to being 'held in mind' by you. It can also be nice to make a larger affirmation card to stick on your child's bedroom wall.

They are the perfect way to teach children their true value and that they're not their feelings or thoughts. This distancing from feelings and thoughts is one of the most powerful ways mindfulness can help children. When mindfulness meets kindfulness, you naturally turn down the brain's negativity in favour of a more balanced perspective and warmth towards yourself and others. What a brilliant way to empower a child and to promote lifelong resilience.

Compassion-based resilience

Researchers are finding the key to a happy and successful life is resilience, that is, being able to rebound in the face of difficulties. And the key to resilience is self-compassion.[155] Multiple studies have found that those who rate highest in self-compassion show a greater degree of emotional resilience.

The word 'resilience' derives from the Latin verb 'to jump back' – or 'bounce-back ability', as some like to call it. But what does it actually mean in practice, and how can you best support your child to become more resilient?

Resilience isn't a fixed trait. When we feel emotionally safe and connected to others, it increases. If we are anxious and isolated, it decreases.[156]

Resilience is like a muscle that a child can only exercise and build up the more they experience stress, with their parents by their side to support them.

Anxiety made simple

Question: Is there a positive side to anxiety?

Answer: Most people see anxiety as being a bad thing, so you may be wondering how anxiety could ever be a good thing.

While we no longer have to run away from predators (thank God for that!), feeling a little bit anxious can actually help us to meet a challenge, like reading out loud in class or playing in a football game.

The adrenaline that gets released when we think there's a threat gives us a big boost of energy, which helps us to do our best.

A lot of people would even say that nerves can sometimes feel quite like excitement! Have you ever felt butterflies in your belly when you're really excited about something? I know I have, and it doesn't feel too different from the butterflies in my belly when I feel anxious.

The big difference between belly butterflies being a good thing and being a bad thing is the way we think about situations. If we have negative, worried thoughts about a challenge, these will make the butterflies feel a lot worse, which in turn will send a message to our brains that something's dangerous.

On the other hand, if we have positive excited thoughts about a challenge, we probably won't really notice the butterflies, or if we do they won't bother us as much, since our attention is focused on the fun thing we're about to do.

So the way we think about a situation makes a huge difference as to whether we see it as a threat or as an opportunity.

This brings me to your superpowers – and you may not realise that you have many of these! I didn't know much about my anxiety superpowers until I grew up, so here's a sneak peek at just some of the things you're sure to be good at:

- *You've got a powerful imagination.* Just like you can imagine things going wrong when you're feeling anxious, you can use your colourful imagination to see situations in new and inventive ways. It's just like a muscle: the more you use it, the more creativity can come from it!

- *You can prepare your body to do its best.* Because you're so aware of how your body feels when you're anxious, your alarming adrenaline can act as your own secret rocket fuel to propel you to think clearly, to lead your way into challenges and even face some of your fears.
- *You're a really good friend.* Your brain is used to scanning for threats, so you'll also be good at scanning into other people's hearts and trying your best to help them. Just be careful not to take on other people's worries too much – and make sure you share your own too.
- *You've got fire in your belly.* Because you're aware of other people's feelings and what's going on for you, you're more likely to show a lot of commitment, care and passion for the things you choose to do in your life. You'll see the fruits of this as you grow older.
- *You're brave.* It's tough being anxious and you've had a lot to deal with. Believe me, this has made you a lot stronger in managing big feelings. There are many things you've overcome in your life already, so high five to you!

Learning to cope with manageable threats is critical for a child developing resilience. Not all stress is harmful, and there are numerous opportunities in every child's life to expose them to positive stresses:

Resilience is something we learn by experiencing stresses. If we never experienced any stresses then it is very difficult for us to learn the methods for dealing with them. For children who are over-protected and only experience good things and success, the evidence is when they reach young adulthood they're emotionally more vulnerable to experiencing pain, because for them stress and anxiety are strange and frightening beasts because they have never experienced them. So we must not mollycoddle our children. They need to be vaccinated against stress the way we are against measles.[157]

Positive stresses can look something like this: letting your child do things that you hadn't let them do previously; giving them plenty of opportunities for free play; not stepping in every time they face a problem; enabling them to negotiate difficult situations by themselves; not shielding them from all pain; reducing excessive reassurance; challenging their negative thoughts; and encouraging them to gradually face their fears. Take your pick!

> When we think of resilience it is often with the idea of it being a skill to endure life's difficulties ... However, the principal driving force of compassion-based resilience is that we remove this idea of seeing problems as problems and more as welcome opportunities to learn and to grow. By doing this we take a kinder approach to ourselves and have more energy to deal with 'the problem'. The essential thing is to turn towards ourselves in times of need and to replace pressure with compassion. This is a skill that needs to be cultivated through repeated practice.[158]

As we know, a child's capacity for self-soothing is born out of repeated instances of being soothed by their parent. Similarly, if a parent encounters stressors as welcome challenges, then their child will show more resilience, whereas if they encounter them as something to run away from or fight against then the child will also struggle to cope. How children and parents think about things has a huge bearing on our ability to bounce back from difficulties.

In helping an anxious child become more compassionately resilient:

> Acknowledge and highlight all their progress. Accept them entirely and love them unconditionally, ensuring that they know that your love is not dependent on any performance or meeting expectations you may have. Shed any expectations of them or yourself and allow them to shine. Allow their greatness to come to the surface through your continual love.[159]

As well as acknowledging our children's progress, it is vitally important to acknowledge our own progress as parents. It's harder to build on something which isn't given due recognition. So I'm asking you to do the following: every time you reflect on yourself, pause and respond to your child's need using a compassionate approach, please give yourself some kindness and encouragement. The more you acknowledge your own strength, the more your child will, which is a win-win all round.

A message of hope for you

And so we come to the end of our journey together. It's been quite the journey, one in which I sincerely hope you have felt warmth and compassion towards the struggles you face.

What you're going through is not easy, and you're trying your very best for your little one. By picking up this book, you've shown how much you want to support your child to navigate the stormy seas of life and anxiety with you by their side. Regardless of *how* you support them and the tools you choose to use, that you *want* to help them is a very promising start. After all, everything grows from the seed of intention.[160]

If nothing else, I hope you've felt a sense of *hope* beaming out through these pages. It's never too late to try something new with your child. Every change that you make for the better, no matter how small, can have a deep impact on their emotional well-being and on the strength of your relationship, which will stand them in good stead well into the future.

Love in, love out

The most precious gift we can give our children is to create a calm and loving environment where they feel safe to feel anxious and are accepted just as they are. Welcome and love all parts of them including their anxiety. We don't have to fix all their problems immediately. The parent who is compassionate to themselves opens the opportunity to be patient with their children. Patience is one of the purest forms of love.[161]

I'm still learning every day to inhale *Love in* to myself so I can exhale *Love out* to my girlies and the world. Hopefully, with practice, it will become more like home to me. My biggest wish for you as a parent is that reading my book has helped you to see the importance of bringing compassion into your relationship with yourself and your child. I'm like you, experiencing all the highs and lows that come with parenting, and trying and trying again. Knowing that you're not alone and that you have some tools will hopefully help you on your journey going forward, so that *Love in* and *Love out* could become a bit more like home to you too.

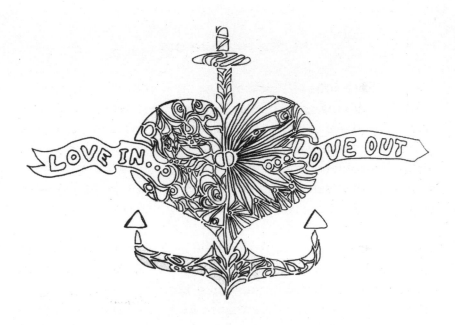

by Caroline Maréchal Brodoux

Appendices

Giving your worry a name[162]

For children aged 4–13

1. Try to come up with a good name for a big worry you have. Paint a picture in your head or on paper of what it looks like.

   Is it big or is it small? What does it say to you? What does its voice sound like? Does it look or sound mean, scary or plain silly?

   Some kids like to think of a worry as a little pest that pops up every now and again just to annoy them, like a worry monster sitting on their shoulder talking into their ear. Seeing a worry as something that isn't part of you can help you feel more control over it.

2. Fill in the blanks with the name you've picked.

3. Sit in a relaxed position or lie down. Close your eyes if you feel comfortable. Place a hand on your belly to make sure you're breathing all the way down into it. If you're lying down, place a soft toy on your belly to check you're breathing deeply into it.

   'The problem is that _____ is calling all the shots but we know that you're really the boss. _____ actually thinks it's protecting you, so what you need to do is let it know that you've got this and that it can relax.

   When you get worried feelings, that means _____ is

*taking over and getting ready to keep you safe. It doesn't
think about it at all, it just jumps in and goes for it.*

What you need to do is to let it know that you're OK.

*One of the best ways to make yourself the boss of your
worry again is breathe. It sounds so simple, and it can be
with practice. Take a deep breath in through your nose and
out through your mouth.*

*Think of something that makes you smile, squeeze your
fingers really tight and breathe.*

*Once your breathing calms, _____ will stop thinking it
has to protect you and will settle back down. Then, quickly
after that, you'll stop feeling the way you do.*

*And breathe. Breathe deeply and slowly. Hold your breath
just for a second between breathing in and breathing out.
Make sure the breath is going right down into your belly,
not just into your chest. You can tell because your belly or
the toy will be moving.*

4. Do this about five to ten times.
5. Practise before bed every day. Remember that _____, the
   warrior part of your brain, has been protecting you for your
   entire life so it might take a little bit of practice to convince
   _____ to chillax a bit.

   *Try talking to your worry and tell it how you really feel. You
   could tell it, 'You're not the boss of me any more.' Keep
   practising and you'll be really good at it in no time. You
   may still see, feel or hear _____ sometimes, but you'll be the
   one in control.'*

Helping your child to cope
with a traumatic event

For parents with children of all ages

Most of us survive in this world by believing it to be a safe place; otherwise we wouldn't set foot outside the door. Traumatic events can shatter this core belief that the world is a safe place, a place that we can rely on. While any traumatic event can leave adults feeling helpless, children are particularly reactive to events that make them feel unsafe.

Based on my experience of working with children and families who have experienced traumatic events in their lives, here is some information on the signs of trauma to look out for and some tips on how to help children to understand and cope following such an event.

Children are actually quite resilient when dealing with traumatic events, but it's good to know the *possible signs* that your child may be experiencing post-traumatic problems, including:

- being anxious, edgy, nervous or agitated

- being aggressive, either verbally or physically

- having flashbacks or repetitive nightmares

- not sleeping in their own bed

- being easily startled by noises or situations similar to the traumatic event

- reverting to younger behaviours such as bed-wetting, nail-biting, thumb-sucking

- finding it difficult to concentrate

- refusing to go to school

- not talking about what happened

- becoming very dependent and clingy

- developing relationship problems with siblings and friends

- undergoing changes in personality

- losing interest and enjoyment in life

If your child displays several of the above symptoms, or if any of them persist for over a month or significantly impact on their functioning, it could be a sign of a traumatic reaction requiring support from a qualified mental health professional at the earliest opportunity for the best outcome.

Furthermore, parents play a pivotal role in navigating their children's understanding of traumatic events and supporting them through any tricky times. As a parent, it's natural to feel trepidation and to find it difficult answering your children's questions, because you may be processing what has happened yourself. Like adults, children need to talk about their feelings.

Top ten tips for supporting your children after a trauma

1. Reassure your children that you'll do everything to keep them and your family safe.
2. Get a sense of what your child already knows about the traumatic event. It's important that parents play an active role in helping them to understand it. Give them an honest but simple explanation about what happened. Adapt your explanation to their age and level of interest. You know your child best.

3. Let children share any worries or fears with you, take their distress seriously and acknowledge their experience as valid for them. Ask your child from time to time how they're feeling about the event and give them permission to talk, as the post-traumatic effects may occur later than you expect. On the other hand, don't dwell unnecessarily on the events or bombard them with questions, as this could raise their anxiety levels.

4. Young children may not have words to describe their feelings, but given the opportunity they may play out the scenes of the traumatic event. You may worry that this is damaging for your child, but playing out their feelings and reactions is likely to help your child to cope better, so allow them to play while showing acceptance of their feelings. Of course limits should be set if the child is playing in a way that's dangerous to themselves or others. Denial of your child's feelings can lead to bigger problems later on.

5. For older children, be available, listen carefully, watch for times when your child is ready to talk, preferably side to side as opposed to face to face, e.g. in the car, during homework, at bedtime. Give honest answers. If you don't know the answer, tell them you'll come back with it. Don't be afraid to show your feelings in front of your children, as it helps them to see that these reactions are normal and can provide good coping models.

6. Children may need more physical contact and cuddles at this time. Don't worry if they want to sleep in your room at night – they may need this extra security for a little while.

7. Try to keep to other normal routines and activities as much as possible: getting a good night's sleep, eating well, going to school, family meals, attendance at clubs, playdates, etc.

8. Limit children's exposure to violent films or TV programmes and news broadcasts. Children do not have the reasoning abilities or coping mechanisms to deal with repeated views

of people in distress, which may be very upsetting for them at this time.

9. If you're feeling overwhelmed, access the support you need to process your own feelings so you can remain emotionally available to your child with what they're going through.

10. Following a traumatic event, it can be quite common for children to develop minor problems such as bed-wetting, stomach pains, concentration difficulties, sleep problems and withdrawal from normal social activities. With parental awareness and support, these problems are usually temporary and resolve in time. If your child is finding it difficult to return to their normal activities or showing persistent signs of trauma after one month, seek the help of a qualified mental health professional.

Suggestions for dedicated playtime

For parents with children of all ages

When?

- Set aside a specific time for 5–15 minutes each day if you can, or else aim for a few times per week. With young kids, short play works better.

- Use a timer, be it an egg timer, oven timer or stopwatch. Include your child in setting the timer and remind them how much time you have at the beginning. Give them 'five-minute' and 'one minute to the end' reminders, as this will help them to feel contained in the playtime.

- Often children have a hard time finishing play, even if you remind them of the time. If your child knows there will be more playtime coming up during the week, this will make it easier. You can also reflect for them how they may be feeling: 'You seem upset that our playtime is over for today. I really enjoyed it too and look forward to our next time, which is …'

- If you have more than one child, try to play with one of them each day and include it on a daily routine chart posted somewhere so you remember.

- Ideally, playing one-to-one is better, but if you have many kids, try two-to-one or a few together and see how this works.

- If for any reason something comes up and you can't make today's playtime, tell your child when you'll do it instead (preferably the next day or soon after).

What?

- Choose toys and games that your child likes, ones that you can both play with together.

- For pre-verbal babies and toddlers, let them show you which toy they want to play with and remove the other ones so they don't get too distracted.

- As younger children (under fives) can be overwhelmed by too many toys and choices, ask them to pick between two options.

- With an older child (ages five to ten), ask them what they would like to play with and then follow their lead. If they do not initiate play themselves, begin to play in a way you know they enjoy, and invite them to join in with you.

- For teenagers, show an interest in what they like doing and spend time doing it with them. Remember, teens are more likely to share what's going on for them when you're sitting side by side rather than face to face.

How?

- Regardless of their age, get down to your child's level and make eye contact. Your child will know you're ready to play when you're sitting on the floor. I find that sitting on the floor also reminds me that this is mammy playtime and stops me getting distracted.

- Look at your child, mirror their body pose, pay lots of attention and participate wholeheartedly for the few minutes you have together. Be in the moment if you can.

- Follow their lead: avoid asking questions and trying to teach them how to play. You're there to enjoy the play with them, not to educate them in that moment.

- To show your child that you're fully present and paying attention, comment on what they're doing or saying, and reflect on how you're both feeling. For example:
  - Describe the toys and their actions: 'You're using lots of colours to paint that house. I see green over here, red for the roof …'
  - Put words to their feelings: 'You seem so excited to have built that big tower' or 'You seem really frustrated that the blocks won't fit into the trailer.'
  - Put words to your feelings too: 'Jumping on this trampoline is so much fun!'
  - Be a good role model by being calm when something is not going to plan, like those blocks not fitting into the trailer: 'They're just not fitting in as you would like them to. I wonder, are there any other ways we could try?'

- Imitate their sounds, actions and feelings, so it helps them to feel understood and gives you a chance to join in – hum a tune if they're humming, clap if they're clapping.

- Show them you're having fun by laughing with them. Use the opportunity to sit close to them and have plenty of physical contact through play-acting, hugs and so on.

- Encourage them in their play rather than correct them. If your child decides to put the beds into the kitchen of the dollhouse, let them. Instead, take an interest and describe what they're doing: 'You've decided they're all going to sleep in there. They seem really tired.'

- When your child asks what you think of their picture, try to avoid saying, 'It's lovely.' Instead, praise them for their creative expression: 'You mixed the red and green to make this, and you've made a huge sun over there.' This will make them less conscious of their performance and more in tune with the joy of creating.

- Describe and praise your child's positive behaviours, such as sharing or turn-taking.

- Finish the playtime by summarising what you did together, how much you enjoyed it and when the next time is.

- Here's a handy acronym for you to remember: **LISTEN**.
  Look at your child's idea
  Imitate what they're doing to show them you notice
  Sit at their level so that you can see each other's faces
  Tell them what's happening by naming what both of you
      are doing
  Enjoy each other and let it show on your face
  Name the feelings you both have at the time.

STOP mindfulness exercise

For parents and teenagers

Creating space in your day to STOP, take stock and get back into the present helps to calm your stress levels and recharge you. Being in the present moment helps you to gain perspective and create space between your thoughts, feelings and behaviours. This perspective leads us to make wiser decisions and kinder choices for ourselves.

Here's a way to check your mental weather that you can weave into your day:

STOP what you're doing. Put things down for a minute.

TAKE a few deep breaths.

OBSERVE your experience just as it is. Connect with how you feel and what you're thinking. Don't judge your thoughts and feelings. Check in with how your body feels. What do you need right now?

PROCEED with something that will nourish you in the moment.

Think about where there are opportunities in the day for you to just STOP – maybe as you're waking up, taking a shower, or before eating a meal, at a traffic light or at work. What would it be like in the days, weeks, and months ahead if you started STOPping more often?

Love in, love out meditation for parents and teenagers

Begin the meditation by sitting or lying down in a comfortable position and sinking into the surface beneath you, allowing yourself to be held, contained and supported.

Come home to your body and notice the feeling of your back being well supported and your feet safely anchored to the earth.

Close your eyes, if you feel comfortable doing so, and begin to filter out the noise and busyness of your day.

Now is your time to relax and get what you need. This is a time for you to let go, to recharge and to look after you.

Notice any internal sensations in your body and remind yourself that you are bringing loving and kind awareness to your experience as you breathe in love … and breathe out love.

If you like, show yourself care by putting both your hands on your heart. Notice how your body reacts to this warm gesture. Feel free to leave your hands on your heart for the meditation, or if you prefer gently rest them on your belly or by your side.

Allow your worries about the day to drift away like a wave creeping away from the shore. You don't need them in this moment. It is also OK to let them go. Let your mind and body rest for a little while.

Begin to notice your breathing in and out of your belly. Become aware of what it's like for your body to breathe in, deeply filling with air … and to breathe out fully, slowly letting it go …

Breathe in through your nose letting your belly expand fully … breathe out through your mouth letting your belly contract slowly. Just notice what it feels like to breathe right now; breathing deep into your nose and breathing out slowly through your mouth.

Now is your time to recharge your batteries and to nurture yourself fully in your breath. Pay attention to your in-breath and give yourself what you need in this moment. If you're struggling with anything in your life, breathe in what you need right now.

Perhaps it is love, understanding, affection, kindness, forgiveness or strength. Whatever it is you feel you need right now, practise breathing it in, with each breath breathing in something good for yourself to nurture the special person that you are.

Breathing love in ... holding it ... and breathing love out ...

Allow yourself to breathe in something good for yourself with each inhalation. Breathing in kindness to yourself, breathing out kindness to others. Breathing in strength to face your struggles, breathing out strength to those who hold a special place in your heart.

Notice how your body feels nourished with the in-breath and relaxes with the out-breath.

Feel the rhythm of your breathing, slowly in and out of your body, helping your mind to empty itself of the worries it doesn't need to hold on to. Feeling calmer, clearer and more nourished with each breath.

When you breathe in, breathe in a feeling of warmth, a deep sense of compassion for yourself and the love of those who mean the most to you. When you breathe out, share the infinite good within you and all of the love and kindness you have to bring to the world.

Give yourself the gift of your breath as you relax further still into the surface beneath you.

Breathing love in ... hold it ... and breathing love out ...

Feel your body moving gently with the in- and the out-breath, like waves coming in and then going back out. In and out. In and out. Like the waves of an ocean. A vast ocean of love, of kindness and of strength.

As you do this, your mind will naturally wander away with your many thoughts. That is all right. When this happens, just notice this without judgement, with love and kindness for yourself and gently return to the beautifully natural rhythm of your breathing.

Try not to judge yourself. You are whole as you are without needing to change anything. You are perfect just as you are in this moment.

You are deeply loved and you love with all your heart.

Allow your whole body to be rocked and nurtured with infinite love by your breath.

Breathing love in … hold it … and breathing love out …

Become your breath; it is your closest ally, always by your side, when you most need it.

Remember you can anchor yourself in this way using your breath any time of the day by breathing love in … and breathing love out.

Keep breathing in and out for a while and feel what it's like to be at one with your breath.

Slowly release your focus on the breath and gently come back into your body. Let yourself feel whatever it is you are feeling in the moment and be just as you are.

There is no right or wrong way to feel; how you feel right now is perfectly OK. You are just right as you are.

Show yourself this love by placing your hands on your heart. Give yourself warmth for today and for always.

And when you're ready, slowly and gently come back into the room feeling calm, nurtured and relaxed. Bring this love and compassion for yourself and others with you as you go through your day.

Slowly open your eyes. Stretch your arms out and back in around your shoulders for a hug.

And finally breathe one last big breath in and a big breath out. Love in … and love out …

Love in, love out kind breathing
meditation for children[163]

When you're ready, lie down. Close your eyes if you like, and put your hands on your belly. Can you feel your belly moving as you breathe in and out? Just notice your belly moving as you breathe in and out. What does it feel like?

Now, imagine that all around you is a beautiful, bright, white light – the most beautiful white light that you have ever seen. Imagine this beautiful, white, glistening light is filled with feelings of kindness, filled up with feelings of kindness. Can you imagine breathing in this beautiful, white, sparkling light? Can you see it filling up your head, your heart, your tummy, your whole body with beautiful feelings of kindness? Filling you up with kindness from the top of your head to the tips of your toes?

Now that you're filled up with kindness, see if you can practise breathing out this bright white light. See if you can breathe out this kindness to your family, friends, to the children in your school, to your neighbours and to the people in your town. See them smile as you breathe out kindness to them. Breathing in kindness for yourself, breathing out kindness for your family. Breathing in kindness for yourself, breathing out kindness for your friends.

Breathing in kindness for yourself, breathing out kindness for your neighbours. How does it feel to breathe in and out kindness?

Now, imagine that all around you is a beautiful, shining, green light, the most beautiful green light that you have ever seen. Imagine this shimmering green light is filled with feelings of friendship, filled up with feelings of friendship. Can you imagine breathing in this beautiful, green, shining light? Can you see it filling up your head, your heart, your tummy, your whole body with feelings of friendship? Filling you up with friendship from the top of your head to the tips of your toes?

Now that you're filled up with friendship, see if you can practise breathing out this bright green light. See if you can breathe out this friendship to your family, friends, to the people you know and to the people you don't know. See them smile as you breathe out friendship to them. Breathing in friendship for yourself, breathing out friendship to your family. Breathing in friendship for yourself, breathing out friendship for your friends. Breathing in friendship for yourself, breathing out friendship to all the children in your school. How does it feel to breathe in and out friendship?

Now, imagine that all around you is a beautiful, glittering, red light, the most beautiful red light that you've ever seen. Imagine this glistening red light is filled with feelings of love, filled up with feelings of love. Can you imagine breathing in this beautiful, glittering, red light? Can you see it filling up your head, your heart, your tummy, your whole body with feelings of love? Filling you up with love from the top of your head to the tips of your toes?

Now that you're filled up with love, see if you can practise breathing out this glittering red light. See if you can breathe out this love to your family, friends, to people who are similar to you and to people who are different to you. See them smile as you breathe out love to them. Breathing in love for yourself, breathing out love for your family. Breathing in love for yourself, breathing out love for your friends, breathing in love for yourself, breathing out love for all the people you know. How does it feel to breathe in and out love?

How do you feel now after breathing in this kindness, friendship and love for yourself? How does it feel to breathe out this kindness, friendship and love to others? Is there anything else you feel you need right now? Maybe it's strength, peace or calm? Before we finish, imagine there's a beautiful rainbow light around you now, and it's filled with everything you need right now, everything you need to feel good and strong inside. Imagine breathing in this beautiful rainbow light and see it filling you up, see it filling you up with everything you need right now from the top of your head to the tips of your fingers and toes. Breathing in good things for yourself!

Now breathe out this beautiful rainbow light to others, to your family and friends, to your neighbours, to the people you know and the people who you don't know. Breathe in rainbow light for yourself and breathe out rainbow light to others. Breathe out this rainbow light to your whole town, to your whole country, and now breathe out the rainbow light to the whole world. Breathing in and breathing out all these good things, breathing in and breathing out all these kind things.

Now it's time to end the meditation. Notice how you feel now. This is how it feels to breathe in kind things for ourselves and others. If you like how it feels, why not practise it as you go through your day. Just breathe in and out kindness, breathe in and out friendship, breathe in and out love. You can do this any time you like!

Now, when you're ready, wriggle your fingers and toes and gently open your eyes.

Bumblebee breath

For children aged 4–13

1. Sit in a comfortable position. Imagine you're a bee sitting on a flower petal. Allow the petal to fully support you.
2. Put your hand on your belly to make sure you're breathing deep into it. Breathe in and out a few times, and feel your belly filling up and relaxing down.
3. Close your eyes if you feel comfortable doing so. Use your fingertips to lightly cover your closed eyelids. Now use your fingers to cover your ears.
4. Breathe in deeply through your nose, filling up your lungs all the way down into your belly.
5. As you breathe out, let out a long, humming sound like a bee for as long as you can: *buzzzzzzzzzzzzzzzzzzzzzzz* … With your eyes and ears closed, you can really hear the sound of the buzzing bee in your head. Let it relax you. Really relax you. See how far your bee flies before resting again.
6. Breathe in again, and as you breathe out, see if you can let out a much louder and stronger buzz this time: *BUZZZZZZZZZZZZZZZZZZZZZZZZ* …
7. Breathe in again, and as you breathe out, see if you can let out a much softer and gentler buzz this time: *buzzzzzzzzzzzzzzzzzzzzzzz* …
8. How does your buzz feel today? Does it feel different with a loud or soft buzz? When you're ready, gently open your eyes and bring your attention back into the room. Get up and shake your body all around!

Follow-up activity

If you and your child like, after breathing practice, draw a picture of a bumblebee and the flower you were sitting on. This picture, or the one you already have in your imagination, can be used as a relaxation practice reminder. When you see the picture, practise buzzing like a bee again: *buzzzzzzzzzzzzzzzzzzzzzzzzz* ...

Why bumblebee breathing works

Bee breathing creates vibrations throughout the body. This is great for showing children the different sensations in their bodies and demonstrating that everything they do has an effect on their body, even breathing. Bumblebee breathing is great because it teaches patience and moderation. If you hum too quickly, you run out of breath faster. But if you take your time and slow your breath, you can hum for a longer time. Bumblebee breathing calms the mind and can inspire new creative ideas. Most of all, it's a *fun* way to practise mindfulness!

The Wheel of Awareness[164]

For children aged 8 and above

Children sometimes need a visual tool to help them tune in to their senses, thoughts, physical sensations and their connection to the world around them.

Photocopy the printable template of the Wheel on page 261, cut out the pieces and stick them on cardboard – children may want to colour in the pictures. Then assemble the wheel with the hub (child meditating) in the middle and the arrow to move around. Use a split pin to connect the parts so the arrow can spin freely.

Go through the wheel with your child the first few times so they can get used to it. After a few trial runs, children can do it independently, and you could encourage them to use it regularly or even practise it together.

1. Start the arrow at the Senses and ask them:
   'What do I hear?' – *tune in to the sounds around you.*
   'What do I see?' – *look around at what you can see.*
   'What do I smell?' – *become aware of any scents.*
   'What tastes are in my mouth?' – *pay attention to your sense of taste.*
   'What can I feel on my skin?' – *focus on the sensations on your skin.*
2. Move the arrow left to the next section, Inner sensations.
   Move your attention inside your body.
   'Can I feel any tingling, discomfort, pain, tension, heat, movement or any other sensation?'
   Become aware of the different parts of your body for a few minutes, from your toes all the way up to the top of your head.

The Wheel of Awareness

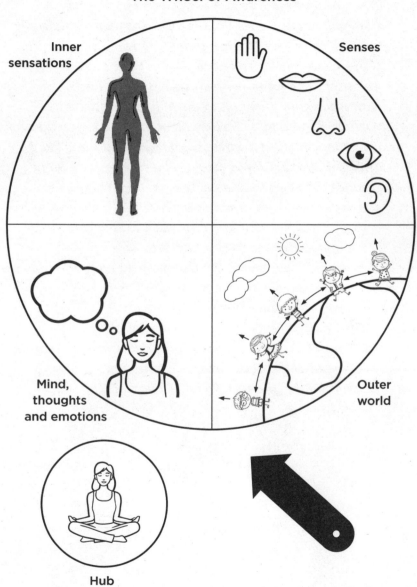

Inner sensations

Senses

Mind, thoughts and emotions

Outer world

Hub

3. Move the arrow to the Mind, thoughts and emotions section.

> *'What am I thinking of?'*
> *'What emotions am I feeling at the moment?'*
> *Think of your mind as a blue sky with passing clouds (thoughts) or as a guesthouse where everybody is welcome, and will come and go when they're ready.*
> *Name or label them and let them go: 'There's a worry; Hello, jealousy; Good morning, gratitude; Bye-bye, anger.'*
> *Now move your attention to the hub (picture of child meditating) and try to include all of the different sections of awareness into just awareness and feel what that's like. This is the most abstract part, and it takes quite a bit of practice. Don't get frustrated. If your mind wanders and you notice it – that's awareness! Our minds will always be active. Just direct your attention back to your breathing again and again whenever it happens.*

4. Finally, move the arrow to the Outer world section, including the people, the room and the environment – basically all our connections to the world.

> *Ask yourself 'Where am I?'; 'Who am I with?'*
> *You can extend your connection to wherever you like, even if it's to our planet Earth and its connections to other planets and the universe. We are all part of 'The One'.*

The Five Ps map

For children of any age, for completion by/with their parent as appropriate (see page 104 for explanations of what each P represents)

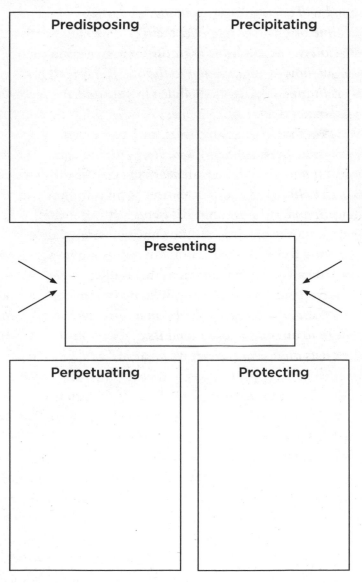

Predisposing	Precipitating

Presenting

Perpetuating	Protecting

Red and green thoughts[165]

For children aged 8 and above

1. Show your child the 'Learning to think green thoughts' example (see page 265) and the explanations of red and green thoughts (see page 121) and go through it with them. Share some examples of your own where a situation provoked both negative red thoughts (unhelpful) and positive green thoughts (helpful) in you, and the feelings and behaviours that arose from each way of thinking and feeling.

2. Move on to the 'Changing unhelpful red thoughts' worksheet (see page 266). Ask your child to think of a difficult situation. Next, ask them to come up with at least one unhelpful red thought for that situation. Ask your child to write down the feelings they had following from that red thought. Then ask them to list the 'behaviours' they displayed following the unhelpful red thoughts and feelings.

3. Ask your child to think of some helpful green thoughts in response to the same situation. Write in the feelings and behaviours that arose from the green thoughts and feelings. Talk to your child about how each way of thinking changed their experience of the same situation.

4. Use everyday opportunities to direct your child's attention to their unhelpful red thoughts. Do this when your child is calm and able to use their problem-solving brain. If your child is having a very anxious moment, anchoring them back to safety works best first.

5. For every unhelpful red thought, ask your child to come up with a more helpful green thought. If your child finds this difficult, give them an example from your own experience that they can understand: 'I could see that I wasn't going to get that job as I was not good enough (unhelpful red

thought); but maybe it wasn't the right job for me, and something better will come up (helpful green thought).'

Learning to think green thoughts

If your child feels uncomfortable, ask them to explain red and green thoughts to others.

Sharing out loud some of your own thoughts can help your child to recognise whether thoughts are helpful or unhelpful, so try to give some appropriate examples from your own experience.

Encourage your child to focus on the positives of any situation and to have realistic green thoughts.

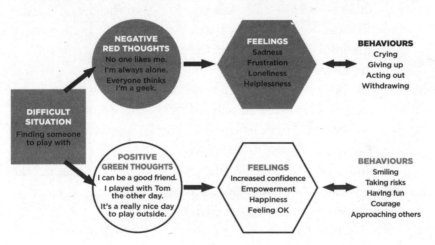

Changing unhelpful red thoughts

Fill in the diagram and learn how to change your thoughts from unhelpful red thoughts to helpful green thoughts.

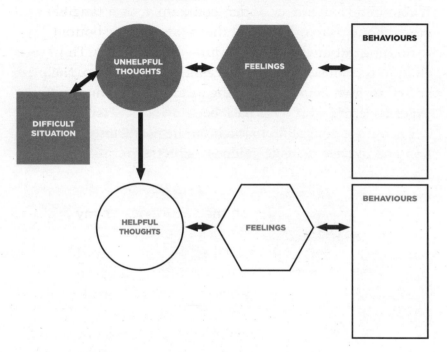

Tom's fear ladder

For children aged 8 and above

When designing a fear ladder, come up with a tangible end goal and put that at the top of the ladder. On the bottom step, write down what the child can just about do now. This helps them to experience a bit of success from the get go. Next, fill in the steps in between, starting at the bottom and working your way up. Most ladders have between six and ten steps. The child can rate their fear for each step if this helps.

Looking at Tom's fear ladder from the bottom to the top, these were the steps:

GOAL: I'll be able to go on the school bus on my own to and from school every day.

On the third week of school, I'll get on the bus myself and my parents won't send a text. My friend will sit nearby if he can. I'll build up going home by bus that week and break down into smaller steps if I need.

On the second week of school, I'll get on the bus myself and my parents will send me a text. My friend will get on the bus and sit close by. My parents will collect me from school.

On the first three days of school, my friend will come to my house and we'll get on the bus to school together and sit close together. My parents will collect me from school.

Before school starts, we'll repeat the bus journey in the car and ask my friend (who's also taking the school bus) to join us for the ride.

START: Before school starts, my parents will drive me to the bus stop, and we'll follow the bus route to school until we reach the school gate, where we can see where I get off.

Useful tips for parents when trying out a fear ladder:

- Get your child involved in planning the ladder so they feel ownership over it. Pick the right time to try out a new step, when you are both in a good frame of mind.

- Make sure you give your child tons of praise for each attempt at a step; even if it doesn't go particularly well, at least they've tried. Give them a small reward after achieving each step, which you can plan in advance and offer as soon as possible.

- Although a fear ladder looks linear, some steps may need to be repeated several times before your child is comfortable moving on. If you feel that the next step is too tough, consider making it a bit easier. It's OK to tweak the steps as you go along.

- To design your own fear ladder, there are some practical tips,[166] examples,[167] and a blank copy available via the links in the Notes.[168]

How to make a worry box

For children aged 4–13

Worries overwhelm us when too many of them get jumbled up in our minds. Asking your child to make a worry box gives them an opportunity to share their worries with you in a safe and contained way, which works to calm their minds from unnecessary worries.

   Suggested steps:

1. Use a shoe box, jar or any other type of container. Some children like to decorate it and really make it their own. If welcomed, don't be afraid to help out yourself!
2. Ask your child to write down a few worries on little pieces of paper. If your child agrees, feel free to write down a few worries you think your child might have. Fold the pieces of paper and put them into the worry box.
3. Ask your child to keep their worry box in a safe place outside their bedroom (e.g. your bedroom, or anywhere discreet).
4. Build worry time into your routine, when you are alone with your child and with few interruptions. Keep a time limit on it, for example 10–15 minutes, which you both allow for a few times a week. When the time is over, move on and explore it further the next time.
5. Make sure to create the emotional space within you to feel calm and able to listen to your child's worries. Show a sense of calm and patience with your body language and words.
6. Ask your child to pick a worry from their worry box and share it with you. If they pick your piece of paper, explain to them what prompted you to write it down (e.g. 'I noticed that you seem to tense up when X happens').
7. Gently discuss the worry with your child and really listen to

what they have to say. Try not to reassure them. Unpack why they may be feeling this way and reflect your understanding back to them. Speaking their worry out loud often takes some of the charge out of it.

8. Ask your child what they think might help with their worry or share your wisdom on what you think may help to ease it. If there is something you can do to help, ask them if this would be all right. Empower your child as much as you can and praise any small brave step.

9. Following your discussion, let your child decide the following: if the worry is no longer a worry, encourage them to tear it up and put it in the bin. If the worry is still a worry, ask them to re-post it into the worry box for another time and rate it, if you like.

10. If it's helpful, ask your child to rate the worry out of ten on the back of the piece of paper, where one is slightly worried and ten is extremely worried. Add the date too so that you can track your child's worries over time and hopefully really see an improvement. Good luck!

Resources

Recommended reading for parents or educators

Based on my clinical work with families, listed below are selected books on anxiety, self-compassion and managing big emotions which may be of interest to parents or educators.

Brennan, F. (2019). *The positive habit: 6 steps for transforming negative thoughts to positive emotions*. Dublin, Ireland: Gill Books.

Cohen, L. (2013). *The Opposite of Worry: The Playful Parenting Approach to Childhood Anxieties and Fears*. New York: Random House.

Foran, C. (2017). *Owning it: Your bullsh*t-free guide to living with anxiety*. Dublin, Ireland: Hachette.

Garber, B. D. (2016). *Holding Tight, Letting Go: Raising Kids in Anxious Times*. Scottsdale, US: HCI.

Hartzell, M., & Siegel, D. J. (2014). *Parenting from the Inside Out: How a Deeper Self-Understanding Can Help You Raise Children Who Thrive*. Carlton North, Australia: Scribe.

Hoffman, K. Cooper, G., Powell, B., & Benton, C. M. (2017). *Raising a Secure Child: How Circle of Security Parenting Can Help You Nurture Your Child's Attachment, Emotional Resilience, and Freedom to Explore*. New York: Guilford.

Knost, L.R. (2013). *Whispers Through Time: Communication Through the Ages and Stages of Childhood*. Orlando, U.S.: Little Heart Books.

Koster, A. (2018). *Roots and Wings: Childhood Needs a Revolution*. Tipperary, Ireland: Roots & Wings Publishing.

Neff, K., & Germer, C. (2018). *The Mindful Self-Compassion Workbook: A Proven Way to Accept Yourself, Build Inner Strength and Thrive*. New York: Guilford.

Siegel, D. J. & Bryson, T. P. (2012). *The Whole Brain Child: 12 Revolutionary Strategies to Nurture Your Child's Developing Mind*. New York: Random House.

Sunderland, M. (2016). *What Every Parent Needs to Know: Love, Nurture and Play with Your Child* (2nd ed.). London: Dorling Kindersley.

Welford, M. (2016). *Compassion Focused Therapy for Dummies*. New York: John Wiley & Sons.

Books for use with children

Below are selected workbooks and children's storybooks for use by parents or educators with children who are experiencing anxiety.

Breslin, N. (2018). *The Magic Moment*. Dublin, Ireland: Gill Books. A nice little mindfulness technique used for managing big feelings for ages 4–8.

Evans, J. (2016). *Little Meerkat's Big Panic: A Story About Learning New Ways to Feel Calm*. London: Jessica Kingsley Publishers. A storybook for ages 4–8 to help children manage feelings of stress, anxiety and panic, including useful brain metaphors.

Forman, F. (2019). *Self-Kindness for Kids: Whizzo-Voice to the Rescue!* Co. Kildare, Ireland: Outside the Box Learning

Resources. Interactive self-help book for children aged eight and over helping them to turn down their critical voice in favour of their kind inner voice.

Huebner, D. (2005). *What to Do When You Worry Too Much: A Kid's Guide to Overcoming Anxiety*. Washington, D.C.: American Psychological Association. An interactive self-help book for ages 6–12 and parents, introducing CBT techniques for generalised anxiety; books in the same series also available on the fear of making mistakes, social anxiety, Obsessive-Compulsive Disorder and separation anxiety.

Huebner, D. (2017). *Outsmarting Worry: An Older Kid's Guide to Managing Anxiety*. London: Jessica Kingsley Publishers. An interactive self-help book for ages 9–13 and their parents, with teenage-friendly tools for anxiety.

Ironside, V. (2011). *The Huge Bag of Worries*. London: Hachette Children's Group. A nice storybook for ages 3–8 on carrying big feelings and the value of sharing them.

Karst, P. (2001). *The Invisible String*. Marina Del Rey, US: DeVorss & Co. A lovely storybook for ages 4–8 with fear of separation fostering the attachment relationship.

Shanagher, L. & Finerty, R. (2018). *Mindfully Me 3-Pack*. Dublin: The Lilliput Press. Amazing series of mindfulness books introducing mindful breathing, kindness and self-compassion for ages 4–8.

Sloane, M. & Del Giudice, V. (2018). *Feathers*. California, US: CreateSpace Independent Publishing Platform. A heartening storybook for ages 4+ that teaches children the importance of feelings, boundaries and self-love.

Stallard, P. (2002). *Think Good – Feel Good: A Cognitive Behaviour Therapy Workbook for Children and Young People*. West Sussex: John Wiley & Sons. A great CBT resource for ages 10+. Available as free PDF online: http://blogs.sch.gr/fmarvel/files/2014/04/Paul_Stallard_Think_Good_-_Feel_Good_.pdf.

Sunderland, M. (2003). *Teenie Weenie in a Too Big World: A Story for Fearful Children*. London: Taylor & Francis. A storybook for ages 5–10 who struggle with worries; storybooks from the same series also available on dealing with general anxiety, OCD and separation anxiety.

Woloshyn, L. (2009). *Mighty Moe: An Anxiety Workbook for Children*. An anxiety workbook for children aged 5–8 and their parents/educators. Available as free PDF online: http://cache.trustedpartner.com/docs/library/MentalHealth PBC2009/Mighty%20Joe%20Workbook.pdf.

Young, K. (2019). *Hey Warrior*. London: New Frontier. A storybook for school-aged children explaining why anxiety feels the way it does, empowering them with strategies.

Zelinger, L. E., & Zelinger, J. (2014). *Please Explain Anxiety to Me!: Simple Biology and Solutions for Children and Parents* (2nd. ed). Ann Arbor, US: Loving Healing Press. A story for ages 5–8 explaining the brain–body connection underlying anxiety.

Workbooks for use with parents

Below are selected workbooks for use by health professionals or educators with parents of children with anxiety.

Cartwright-Hatton, S., Laskey, B., Rust, S., McNally, D. (2010). *From Timid to Tiger: A Treatment Manual for Parenting the Anxious Child*. Hoboken, US: John Wiley A treatment manual for therapists for use with parents of anxious children aged ten and below.

Creswell, C., & Willetts, L. (2007). *Overcoming Your Child's Fears and Worries: A Self-Help Guide Using Cognitive Behavioural Techniques*. London: Little, Brown. A self-help treatment guide that enables parents of 5– 12-year-olds to

understand the factors contributing to their child's
worries, offering practical strategies to help them.

Siegel, D. J. & Bryson, T. P. (2015). *The Whole Brain Child
Workbook: Practical Exercises, Worksheets and Activities to
Nurture Developing Minds.* Minneapolis, US: Blue Book.
A workbook with applications for parents, clinicians,
educators and caregivers.

Sunderland, M. (2003). *Helping Children with Fear: A
Guidebook.* London: Taylor & Francis. Accompanies the
same author's *Teenie Weenie in a Too Big World*, for ages
5–10. Guidebooks are also available to accompany
storybooks on general anxiety, OCD and separation anxiety.

Recommended websites

*Here are my favourite websites that I most recommend in my
work with children and families.*

www.alustforlife.com. Irish movement for well-being very
close to my heart, including articles by professionals and
personal stories of mental health struggles and journeys of
recovery.

www.anxietycanada.com. Brilliant website with lots of self-
help and evidence-based resources on anxiety and anxiety
disorders, which I often use in explaining the mechanics
of anxiety. Also includes the MindShift™ App and 'My
Anxiety Plan' online course.

www.brendacassidy.com. Occupational therapist, sensory
educator and the developer of the Braincalm Program,
with specially designed activities for children with sensory
issues, autism, ADHD, anxiety and behavioural issues to
help their sense of calm, their overall emotional and
physical regulation, and their readiness for learning.

www.drmaliecoyne.ie. For more of my print, radio and TV work, have a look at my website.

www.getselfhelp.co.uk. Simple CBT (cognitive-behaviour therapy) and DBT (dialectical-behaviour therapy) self-help and therapy resources, including information sheets, worksheets and self-help mp3s.

www.gozen.com. Engaging anxiety-relief techniques for children, including blogs, video animations and programmes on anxiety/stress relief, well-being and resilience, OCD relief, mindfulness, negative thoughts and panic attacks. Try the free masterclass: '9 techniques every parent with an anxious child should try to melt away their anxiety'.

www.heysigmund.com. Psychologist and author Karen Young, which features accessible articles on child anxiety and parenting. Impressive selection of anxiety videos for kids on: https://www.heysigmund.com/category/with-kids/anxiety-videos-for-kids/.

www.louiseshanagher.com. Children's therapist, mindfulness teacher, psychology lecturer, and co-creator of Lou Lou Rose, which aims to nurture and promote positive mental health through her series of *Mindfully Me* books, guided meditation CDs and affirmation cards.

www.rootsandwings.pub. Teacher, author, mum and mindfulness practitioner, with a blog, mindful games and free resources helping parents and educators to promote mindfulness.

www.weavingwellbeing.com. Positive mental health and well-being programme for ages 8–12, including teacher manuals, student activity books, blogs and videos.

Online resources and meditations

https://www.alustforlife.com/mental-health/exam-stress-management-course/a-lust-for-life-exam-stress-management-course-week-1-mastering-the-game-of-exams. My five-week holistic well-being 'Exam Stress Management Course' for students and parents alike.

https://maps.anxietycanada.com/courses/child-map. Free online ten-hour course for parents to coach anxious children and teenagers using anxiety-management tools (e.g. understanding my anxiety, calming strategies, helpful thinking, facing fears, etc.).

http://www.cci.health.wa.gov.au/resources/consumers.cfm. Excellent InfoPax on various mental health issues, including online modules on worries, generalised anxiety disorders, panic attacks, social anxiety, health anxiety, facing your feelings and self-compassion.

https://www.mentalhealth.org.uk/sites/default/files/anxious_child.pdf. A booklet for parent and carers wanting to know more about anxiety in children and young people.

https://www.netmums.com/support/the-compassionate-mind-approach. Much recommended 'mind training' if you want to delve into the treasure trove of compassion-focused therapy.

http://self-compassion.org/category/exercises/#exercises. Guided meditations and compassion-based exercises by Dr Kristin Neff.

Loving Kindness Meditation for Children: Sky Like Mind. By Louise Shanagher. A six-minute loving kindness meditation for kids video. https://www.youtube.com/watch?v=pOE6V6o2y-4&feature=youtu.be.

Body Scan Children's Meditation: Sky Like Mind. By Louise Shanagher. A six-minute body scan meditation for kids video. https://www.youtube.com/watch?v=ShTP0Omzkd4

Children's Fish Pond Meditation for Children: Sky Like
Mind. By Louise Shanagher. a seven-minute awareness
meditation for kids video. https://www.youtube.com/
watch?v=1F5M2hbZOz0

Useful apps for children's anxiety and emotional regulation[169]

*These apps are a great tool for parents and teachers to guide
children through developmentally appropriate mindfulness and
breathing exercises.*

Headspace (for kids). Provides guided meditations on
calmness, kindness and bedtime, which helps children
improve their focus while relieving anxiety and stress.
Suitable for all levels, the app is customised for three age
groups – under 5 years, 6–8 years and 9–12. Teens and
parents can use the adult version to practise mindfulness
alongside the younger child.

Stop, Breathe, and Think Kids. Offers children a playful and
interactive way to discover and develop their superpowers
of sleep, being calm, learning to breathe and resolving
conflicts. Kids can choose from a range of emojis to
represent how they're feeling, which produces customised
activities (mindful missions and meditations) tuned to
those emotions. Largely aimed at children aged 5–10.

Smiling Mind. Developed by psychologists and educators
and designed to help children with the stresses of everyday
life. It has different programs depending on age. This app
has great body-scan meditations, mindfulness, relaxation,
breathing and guided imagery exercises ranging from 2–15
minutes. It also has a section on 'Mindfulness in the
Classroom'.

Notes

1. Siegel, D.J. and Bryson, T.P., *The Whole Brain Child: 12 Revolutionary Strategies to Nurture Your Child's Developing Mind*, Random House, New York, (2012) page ix.
2. Neff, K., 'The newest parenting skill: Self-compassion', Seleni.org, https://www.seleni.org/advice-support/2018/3/21/the-newest-parenting-skill-self-compassion.
3. *Love in, love out* is also reminiscent of the good intentions cultivated by compassionate Loving-Kindness Meditations which reduce negative emotions like anxiety and depression and lead to more supportive self-talk and better moods. Neff's 'Breathing compassion in and out' guides us to nurture themselves with a quality we need with our in-breath (e.g. 'kindness, love'), and to use our out-breath to send compassion to someone who is struggling (e.g. our child). Almost like a parent-child dance of compassion. Neff, K., 'Breathing compassion in and out', Mindful.org, (2018), https://www.mindful.org/breathing-compassion-in-and-out/.
4. Dr Paul D'Alton, principal clinical psychologist at St Vincent's University Hospital, Dublin, gave a compelling radio interview in which he shared why self-compassion is so important. I have adapted Paul's recommended steps to apply to the experience of parents. D'Alton, P., 'Compassion … is best understood as a verb, it's something we do', RTÉ Radio 1 highlights, (2108), https://www.radio.rte.ie/radio1highlights/compassion-drivetime/.
5. If you want to try something like this for yourself, try the grounding five-minute audio 'Self-Compassion Break' – Neff, K., 'Self-compassion break', Self-Compassion.org, (2015) https://self-compassion.org/wp-content/uploads/2015/12/self-compassion.break_.mp3.
6. Neff, K., *Self-compassion: Stop Beating Yourself Up and Leave Insecurity Behind*, Hodder & Stoughton, London, (2011).
7. The dangers of self-criticism were highlighted in my recent contribution to *The Little Book of Sound*, which encouraged readers to become aware of the content and tone of their internal dialogue. Breslin, N., Coyne, M. and Quirke, S., *The Little Book of Sound*, A Lust for Life, Dublin, (2017), page 10.
8. From compassion advocate Dr Róisín Joyce, lead clinical psychologist with the Evidence-Based Therapy Centre, Galway, Ireland.
9. RTÉ 1 *Stressed, From CBT to CFT: Therapy Explained by the Pros*, RTÉ Lifestyle, (2018) https://www.rte.ie/lifestyle/living/2018/0524/965719-from-cbt-to-cft-therapy-explained-by-the-pros/. See page 56 in the 'Parents' chapter for more details.
10. Neff, K., *Self Compassion: Stop Beating Yourself Up and Leave Insecurity Behind*, Hodder & Stoughton, London, (2011) chapter 4.

11. Welford, M., *Compassion Focused Therapy for Dummies*, John Wiley & Sons, West Sussex, UK, (2016), page 12.
12. MacBeth, A. and Gumley, A., 'Exploring Compassion: A meta-analysis of the association between self-compassion and psychopathology', *Clinical Psychology Review*, (2012) 32, pages 545–552.
13. Raes, F., 'Rumination and worry as mediators of the relationship between self-compassion and depression and anxiety', *Personality and Individual Differences*, (2010), 48, pages 757–761.
14. Lowenthal, M., '16 compassion focused therapy training exercises and worksheets, *Positive Psychology*, (2019), https://positivepsychology.com/compassion-focused-therapy-training-exercises-worksheets/.
15. Lowenthal, M. '16 compassion focused therapy training exercises and worksheets, *Positive Psychology*, (2019), https://positivepsychology program.com/compassion-focused-therapy-training-exercises-worksheets/.
16. Compassion focused therapy (CFT) is a type of psychotherapy which integrates techniques from CBT, Person Centered, Gestalt and Narrative therapies with ideas from evolutionary psychology, biology, social psychology, developmental psychology, Buddhist psychology and neuroscience. Gilbert, Paul 'Introducing compassion-focused therapy', *Advances in Psychiatric Treatment*, (2009) 15(3), pages 199–208.
17. Alcoholics Guide, 'Compassion-focused therapy', Inside the Alcoholic Brain.com, (2016), https://insidethealcoholicbrain.com/2016/03/07/compassion-focused-therapy/.
18. Wickremasinghe, N., 'It's not my fault but it is my problem: The role of self-compassion in a VUCA world', (2017), Linkedin, https://www.linkedin.com/pulse/its-my-fault-problem-role-self-compassion-vuca-world-wickremasinghe.
19. Neff, K., 'The physiology of self-compassion', Self-Compassion.org, http://self-compassion.org/the-physiology-of-self-compassion/.
20. A test to show you how self-compassionate you are can be found here: Neff, K., 'Test how self-compassionate you are', Self-Compassion.org, https://self-compassion.org/test-how-self-compassionate-you-are/.
21. Neff, K., 'The chemicals of care: How self-compassion manifests in our bodies', Self-Compassion.org, https://self-compassion.org/the-chemicals-of-care-how-self-compassion-manifests-in-our-bodies/.
22. Ibid.
23. McGonigal, K., 'How to make stress your friend', (2013) TED Global.
24. Bowlby, J., *Attachment and Loss: Vol. 1. Loss*. Basic Books, New York, (1969).
25. 'The Baby Friendly Hospital Initiative (BFHI) is a global campaign by the World Health Organization and the United Nations Children's Fund (UNICEF) which recognises that implementing best practice in the maternity service is crucial to the success of programmes to promote breastfeeding. http://www.babyfriendly.ie/.
26. Coyne, M., 'How to build a happy baby, RTÉ Brainstorm, (2018), https://www.rte.ie/brainstorm/2018/0306/945352-how-to-build-a-happy-baby/.
27. UNICEF UK, 'Building a happy baby: A guide for parents', (2013), https://www.unicef.org.uk/babyfriendly/wp-content/uploads/sites/2/2018/04/happybaby_leaflet_web.pdf.
28. McGonigal, K., 'How to transform stress into courage and connection', *Greater Good Magazine*, (2015). https://www.greatergood.berkeley.edu/article/item/how_to_transform_stress_courage_connection.

29. Gilbert, P., 'Introducing compassion focused therapy', Compassionatemind.co.uk, https://www.compassionatemind.co.uk/uploads/files/introduction-to-compassion-focussed-therapy.pdf.
30. Cohen, L., *The Opposite of Worry: The Playful Parenting Approach to Childhood Anxieties and Fears*, Ballantine Books, Random House, New York, (2013).
31. Other conditions also make anxiety more likely such as Autism Spectrum Disorder; sensory processing difficulties; or children who present with physical disabilities or medical problems.
32. American Psychiatric Association, *Diagnostic and Statistical Manual of Mental Disorders (DSM-5)*, American Psychiatric Publishing, Arlington, USA, (2013), Section II.
33. Vivyan, C., *Anxiety*, Get Self Help, adapted from https://www.getselfhelp.co.uk/docs/AnxietySelfHelp.pdf.
34. Hayes, C., '10 Steps to Help Manage Your Anxiety', *Irish Independent*, (2017)
35. Cannon, M., Coughlan, H., Clarke, M., Harley, M. and Kelleher, I., (2013) *The Mental Health of Young People in Ireland: A Report of the Psychiatric Epidemiology Research across the Lifespan (PERL) Group*, Dublin: Royal College of Surgeons in Ireland, (2013).
36. Wickremasinghe, N., 'It's not my fault but it is my problem: The role of self-compassion in a VUCA world', (2017), Linkedin, https://www.linkedin.com/pulse/its-my-fault-problem-role-self-compassion-vuca-world-wickremasinghe.
37. Brown, B., *Daring Greatly: How the Courage to be Vulnerable Transforms the Way We Live, Love, Parent, and Lead*, Gotham Books, New York, (2012).
38. McLuhan, M. and Fiore, Q., *The Medium is the Massage*, Penguin, London, (1967).
39. Breslin, N., Coyne, M. and Quirke, S., *The Little Book of Sound*. A Lust for Life, Dublin, (2017) page 30.
40. Festinger, L., *A Theory of Social Comparison Processes*, Bobbs-Merrill, Indiana, US, (1954).
41. St. Patrick's Mental Health Service, *World Mental Health Day School Special Programme – Part 1*, https://www.mixcloud.com/SPMHS/world-mental-health-day-school-special-programme-part-1/.
42. Baucells, M. and Sarin, R., *Engineering Happiness: A New Approach for Building a Joyful Life*, University of California Press, Berkeley, US, (2012).
43. https://www.alustforlife.com/mental-health/exam-stress-management-course/exam-stress-management-course-week-5-top-tips-for-bringing-my-own-game.
44. Quinlan, Á., 'Schoolflakes? The children not going to school ... because they don't like it', *Irish Times*, (2018)
45. Kelly, Dr Ciara 2017, 'Has Ireland's overly indulgent softly, softly parenting approach left our kids short changed?', Irish Independent, https://www.independent.ie/life/family/parenting/dr-ciara-kelly-has-irelands-overly-indulgent-softly-softly-parenting-approach-left-our-kids-short-changed-35460218.html.
46. Sharry, J., 'Anxious parents can produce anxious children, so take a breath', *Irish Times*, (2017).
47. Coyne, M., 'Glossing over anxiety will not make it go away – How to empower your child to deal with the stresses of the back-to-school period', *Irish Independent*, (2019)
48. Slade, A., 'Parental reflective functioning: An introduction', *Attachment and Human Development*, (2005), 7(3), pages 269–282.

49. Hartzell, M. and Siegel, D.J., *Parenting From the Inside Out: How a Deeper Self-understanding Can Help You Raise Children Who Thrive*, Scribe, Australia, (2014) page 1.
50. Fonagy, P., Steele, M., Steele, H., Higgitt, A. and Target, M., 'The Emanuel Miller Memorial Lecture 1992: The theory and practice of resilience', *Child Psychology and Psychiatry and Allied Disciplines*, (1994), 35(2), pages 231–257.
51. Hartzell, M. and Siegel, D.J., *Parenting From the Inside Out: How a Deeper Self-understanding Can Help You Raise Children Who Thrive*, Scribe, Australia, (2014) page 5.
52. Hoffman, K., Cooper, G., Powell, B. and Benton, C.M., *Raising a Secure Child: How Circle of Security Parenting can Help You Nurture Your Child's Attachment, Emotional Resilience, and Freedom to Explore*, Guilford, New York, (2017) page 115.
53. Adapted from Hoffman, K., Cooper, G., Powell, B. and Benton, C.M., *Raising a Secure Child: How Circle of Security Parenting can Help You Nurture Your Child's Attachment, Emotional Resilience, and Freedom to Explore*, Guilford, New York, (2017) page 144.
54. Hoffman, K., Cooper, G., Powell, B. and Benton, C.M., *Raising a Secure Child: How Circle of Security Parenting can Help You Nurture Your Child's Attachment, Emotional Resilience, and Freedom to Explore*, Guilford, New York, (2017) page 128.
55. Ibid., page 1.
56. A lovely woman I work with, Patricia Molloy, now a granny, shared this with me.
57. Tartakovsky, M., '5 tips for teaching your kids self-compassion', PsychCentral.com, (2018) https://psychcentral.com/blog/5-tips-for-teaching-your-kids-self-compassion/.
58. Doyle Melton, G., 'First the pain, then the rising', Oprah Winfrey Network: SuperSoul sessions, (2017), https://www.youtube.com/watch?v= BpBnGHjda14.
59. Young, K., 'Anxiety in children: A metaphor to put you in their shoes (and right beside them)', Hey Sigmund.com, https://www.heysigmund.com/anxiety-children-metaphor-put-shoes-right-beside.
60. Ibid.
61. Evans, J., *Little Meerkat's Big Panic: A Story About Learning New Ways to Feel Calm*, Jessica Kingsley Publishers, London, (2016).
62. Ironside, V., *The Huge Bag of Worries*, Hachette Children's Group, London, (2011).
63. Welford, M., *Compassion Focused Therapy for Dummies*, John Wiley & Sons, West Sussex, UK, (2016), page 66.
64. Payne, K.J., *Simplicity Parenting: Using the Extraordinary Power of Less to Raise Calmer, Happier, and More Secure Kids*, Random House, New York, (2010).
65. Ibid., page 8.
66. Ibid., page 10.
67. Gillett, T., 'Simplifying childhood may protect against mental health issues', Raised Good.com, (2016), https://raisedgood.com/extraordinary-things-happen-when-we-simplify-childhood/.
68. Scott, M. and Buck, P.E., 'The town mouse and the country mouse', *The Big Book of Aesop's Fables*, Comlan Publications, (2009) page 3.
69. Doran, J., 'Positive education for the 21st century', (2018), retrieved from TEDx, https://www.youtube.com/watch?v=AdAkyHEYsxY.

70. Byrne, K., 'Tired but wired: Living with anxiety', *Irish Independent*, (2018).
71. Kreps, S., 'Want happier, calmer kids? Simplify their world', *Green Child Magazine*, (2020), https://www.greenchildmagazine.com/simplify-for-happier-calmer-kids/.
72. Payne, K.J., 'Discipline and the four pillars of simplicity'. An excerpt from *The Soul of Discipline: The Simplicity Parenting Approach to Warm, Firm, and Calm Guidance – From Toddlers to Teens*, Ballantine Books, New York, (2015).
73. Neill, M., 'The point of the Three Principles', MichealNeill.org, (2017), https://www.michaelneill.org/cfts1093/.
74. Barrett, P., *Friends for Life Activity Book for Children* (6th Ed.), Barrett Resources Pty., Australia, (2012).
75. Creswell, C. and Willetts, L., *Overcoming Your Child's Fears and Worries: A Self-help Guide Using Cognitive Behavioural Techniques*, Little, Brown Book Group, London, (2007), page 3.
76. Gilbert, P., 'The origins and nature of compassion focused therapy', *British Journal of Clinical Psychology*, (2014), 53, pages 6–41.
77. Welford, M. and Langmead, K., 'Compassion-based initiatives in educational settings', *Educational and Child Psychology*, (2015), 32(1), pages 71–80.
78. Byrne, K., 'Tired but wired: Living with anxiety', *Irish Independent*, (2018).
79. Chris Winson, dad, mental health author and creator of #365daysof compassion.
80. Brown, B., *Daring Greatly: How the Courage to be Vulnerable Transforms the Way we Live, Love, Parent and Lead*, Penguin, London, (2015), page 217.
81. Ibid., page 219.
82. Siegel, D.J. and Bryson, T.P., *The Whole Brain Child: 12 Revolutionary Strategies to Nurture Your Child's Developing Mind*, Random House, New York, (2012), page ix.
83. Perry, B., 'The Three R's: Reaching the learning brain', Beacon House.org, https://beaconhouse.org.uk/wp-content/uploads/The-Three-Rs.pdf. This ties in nicely with the Brain State Models priorities as developed by Bailey, B. A., *Conscious discipline: Building resilient classrooms*, Loving Guidance, (2015)
84. Nicole McGuigan is a social worker, family support worker and chairperson of the Galway Parent Network. Her masters thesis was entitled: 'Exploring social support for mothers during the transition to motherhood', NUIG, (May 2016).
85. Hoffman, K., Cooper, G., Powell, B. and Benton, C.M., *Raising a Secure Child: How Circle of Security Parenting can Help You Nurture Your Child's Attachment, Emotional Resilience, and Freedom to Explore*, Guilford, New York, (2017), page 42.
86. Doyle, G., *Carry on Warrior: The Power of Embracing your Messy, Beautiful Life*, Scribner, New York, (2014), page 291.
87. Hanh Nhat, Thich, *No Mud No Lotus*, Parallax Press, Berkeley USA, (2015).
88. Dr. Roisin Joyce, lead clinical psychologist, Evidence-Based Therapy Centre, Galway, Ireland.
89. Netmums, 'The compassionate mind approach', Netmums.com, (2016), https://www.netmums.com/support/the-compassionate-mind-approach.
90. Garber, B.D., *Holding Tight, Letting Go: Raising Kids in Anxious Times*, HCI, Scottsdale, USA, (2016), page 7.
91. Ibid, page 25.

92. Hoffman, K., Cooper, G., Powell, B. and Benton, C.M., *Raising a Secure Child: How Circle of Security Parenting can Help You Nurture Your Child's Attachment, Emotional Resilience, and Freedom to Explore*, Guilford, New York, (2017), page 63.

93. Bradshaw, M., 'What a "safe person" is and how to become your own', Maliayoga.com, (2017), https://maliayoga.com/2017/03/29/what-a-safe-person-is-and-how-to-become-your-own/.

94. Karst, P., *The Invisible String*, DeVorss & Co, CA, USA, (2001), page 8.

95. Cohen, L., *The Opposite of Worry: The Playful Parenting Approach to Childhood Anxieties and Fears*, Random House, New York, (2013), page 64.

96. Many of the exercises below hail from Cohen's book chapter on 'Relaxation and Roughhousing'. Cohen, L. *The Opposite of Worry: The Playful Parenting Approach to Childhood Anxieties and Fears*, Random House, New York, (2013), pp 62–96.

97. Artigas, L. and Jarero, I., *The Butterfly Hug Protocol*, (2012), https://www.emdrhap.org/content/wp-content/uploads/2014/07/X-I_THE-BUTTERFLY-HUG-PROTOCOL-SEPTEMBER-2012.pdf.

98. Here's a short video on it: Young, K., 'How to calm anxiety using Figure 8 Breathing' (A video for kids), Hey Sigmund.com, https://www.heysigmund.com/how-to-calm-anxiety-using-figure-8-breathing/.

99. Vivyan, C., *Therapy Metaphors*, Getselfhelp.co.uk, (2009), https://www.getselfhelp.co.uk/docs/Metaphors.pdf.

100. Siegel, D. J., *Mindsight: The New Science of Personal Transformation*, Random House, New York, (2010), page 29.

101. Brown, B., 'The power of vulnerability', RSA, (2015), https://www.youtube.com/watch?v=sXSjc-pbXk4.

102. Brown, B., 'Brené Brown on empathy', RSA Short, (2013), https://www.youtube.com/watch?time_continue=12&v=1Evwgu369Jw&feature=emb_logo.

103. Siegel, D.J. and Bryson, T.P., *The Whole Brain Child: 12 Revolutionary Strategies to Nurture your Child's Developing Mind*, Random House, New York, (2012), page 22.

104. Siegel, D.J. and Bryson, T.P., *The Whole Brain Child: 12 Revolutionary Strategies to Nurture your Child's Developing Mind*, Random House, New York, (2012), page 24.

105. Young, K., 'Anxiety in children and teens: How to find calm and courage during anxiety – What all parents need to know', Hey Sigmund.com, https://www.heysigmund.com/anxiety-in-children-anxiety-in-teens/.

106. Winnicott, D. W., *The Child, the Family, and the Outside World*, Penguin Books, (1973), page 17.

107. Siegel, D.J. and Bryson, T.P., *The Whole Brain Child: 12 Revolutionary Strategies to Nurture your Child's Developing Mind*, Random House, New York, (2012), page ix.

108. Sunderland, M., *Using Storytelling as a Therapeutic Tool with Children*, Speechmark, UK, (2000), page xi.

109. Siegel, D.J. and Bryson, T.P., *The Whole Brain Child: 12 Revolutionary Strategies to Nurture your Child's Developing Mind*, Random House, New York, (2012). This is one of Siegel and Bryson's emotional regulation strategies called 'Name it to tame it: Telling stories to calm big emotions', page 29.

110. Young, K., 'Phobias and fears in children – Powerful strategies to try', Hey Sigmund.com, https://www.heysigmund.com/phobias-and-fears-in-children/.

111. Sunderland, M., *Teenie Weenie in a Too Big World: A Story for Fearful Children*, Taylor & Francis, London, (2003)
112. Sunderland, M., *Using Storytelling as a Therapeutic Tool with Children*, Speechmark, UK, (2000), page 17.
113. Siegel, D.J. and Bryson, T.P., *The Whole Brain Child: 12 Revolutionary Strategies to Nurture your Child's Developing Mind*, Random House, New York, (2012), page 79.
114. Hoffman, K., Cooper, G., Powell, B. and Benton, C.M., *Raising a Secure Child: How Circle of Security Parenting can Help you Nurture your Child's Attachment, Emotional Resilience, and Freedom to Explore*, Guilford, New York, (2017), page 128.
115. Siegel, D. J., *Mindsight: The New Science of Personal Transformation*, Random House, New York, (2010), page 1.
116. Landreth, G. and Bratton, S., 'Play therapy', *ERIC Digest*, Greensboro, NC: ERIC Clearinghouse on Counseling and Student Services, (1999), https://www.counseling.org/resources/library/ERIC%20Digests/99-01.pdf. page 1.
117. Fredrickson, B., 'The value of positive emotions' *American Scientist*, (2003), 91, pages 330–335.
118. Cohen, L., 'Playing with anxiety', Hand in hand parenting.com, https://www.handinhandparenting.org/article/dr-lawrence-cohen-playing-anxiety/.
119. Hoffman, K., Cooper, G., Powell, B. and Benton, C.M., *Raising a Secure Child: How Circle of Security Parenting can Help you Nurture your Child's Attachment, Emotional Resilience, and Freedom to Explore*, Guilford, New York, (2017), page 73.
120. Elkind, D., *The Power of Play: Learning What Comes Naturally*, Da Capo Press, New York, (2007), page xvii.
121. 'Outdoor play', *Play and Playground Encyclopaedia*, https://www.pgpedia.com/o/outdoor-play.
122. Gray, P., 'The decline of play and the rise of psychopathology in children and adolescents', *American Journal of Play*, (2011), 3(4), pages 443–463.
123. Ibid.
124. Gray, P., 'The decline of play and rise in children's mental disorders', Psychology Today.com, (2010), https://www.psychologytoday.com/us/blog/freedom-learn/201001/the-decline-play-and-rise-in-childrens-mental-disorders.
125. Coyne, M., *The importance of playgrounds in child development*, Rollercoaster.ie, (2016), https://www.rollercoaster.ie/Article/Your-child-s-development/the-importance-of-playgrounds-in-child-development.
126. Entin, E., *All work and no play: Why your kids are more anxious, depressed*, The Atlantic.com, (2011), https://www.theatlantic.com/health/archive/2011/10/all-work-and-no-play-why-your-kids-are-more-anxious-depressed/246422/.
127. Siegel, D.J. and Bryson, T.P., *The Whole Brain Child: 12 Revolutionary Strategies to Nurture your Child's Developing Mind*, Random House, New York, (2012), page 57.
128. Landreth, G. and Bratton, S., 'Play therapy'. *ERIC Digest*. Greensboro, NC: ERIC Clearinghouse on Counselling and Student Services, (1999), https://www.counseling.org/resources/library/ERIC%20Digests/99-01.pdf.
129. Angelou, Maya, *I Know Why the Caged Bird Sings*, Little, Brown Book Group, London, (1969), Chapter 18.
130. Schaefer, C. E. and Drewes, A. A., 'Play-based approaches for treating childhood anxieties' In A.A. Drewes and C.E. Schaefer (Eds.), *Play-based*

Interventions for Childhood Anxieties, Fears and Phobias, Guilford, New York, (2018), https://www.guilford.com/excerpts/drewes.pdf, page 7.

131. Jennings, S., *Embodiment-Projection-Role (EPR)*, (2002), http://www. suejennings.com/epr.html.

132. Grave, J. and Blisset, J., 'Is cognitive behaviour therapy developmentally appropriate for young children?: A critical review of the evidence', *Clinical Psychology Review*, (2004), 24, pages 399–420.

133. Drewes, A. A. and Schaefer, C.E., (Eds.) 'Play therapy in middle childhood', *American Psychological Association*, Washington DC, (2016), page 3.

134. Bratton, S.C., Landreth, G. L., Kellam, T. and Blackard, S.R., *Child Parent Relationship Therapy (CPRT) Treatment Manual: A 10 Session Filial Therapy Model for Training Parents*, Taylor & Francis, New York, (2006), Session 9.

135. Pransky, J. and Kahofer, A., *What is a Thought (A Thought is a lot)*, Social Thinking, California, USA, (2011), page 2.

136. Creswell, C. and Willetts, L., *Overcoming your child's fears and worries: A self-help guide using Cognitive Behavioural Techniques*. Little, Brown Book Group, London, UK, (2007), page 33.

137. Pamela Carroll Mannion is an accredited Cognitive Behavioural Psychotherapist with 18 years' experience working both in CAMHS and in Student Counselling in NUIG. She currently works in private practice in Galway, Ireland.

138. 'Thinking errors', Therapist Aid.com (2018), https://www.therapistaid.com/ worksheets/cbt-thinking-errors.pdf.

139. Smith, A., 'Why I teach mindfulness to kids', A Lust for Life.com, https:// www.alustforlife.com/mental-health/mindfulness/why-i-teach-mindfulness-to-kids.

140. Koster, A., *Roots and Wings: Childhood Needs a Revolution*. Roots & Wings Publishing, Ireland, (2018), page 55.

141. Welford, M., *Compassion Focused Therapy for Dummies*, John Wiley & Sons, New York, (2016), page 133.

142. Miners, R., 'Collected and connected: Mindfulness and the early adolescent', *Dissertations Abstracts International: Section B. The Sciences and Engineering*, (2008), 68, page 9.

143. Siegel, D. J., 'Wheel of awareness', Wheel of Awareness.com, https://www. wheelofawareness.com/.

144. Koster, A., *Roots and Wings: Childhood Needs a Revolution*, Roots & Wings Publishing, Ireland, (2018), page 201.

145. Louise Shanagher holds a BA and MSc in Psychology and further qualifications in Psychotherapy, Play Therapy and Mindfulness.

146. Shanagher, L. and Finerty, R., *Mindfully Me 3-Pack*, The Lilliput Press, Dublin, (2018).

147. Shanagher, L. and Finerty, R. *It's always there. Mindfully Me Book 1*, The Lilliput Press, Ireland, (2018).

148. Volunteer Ireland 'The impact of volunteering on the health and wellbeing of the volunteer', *Volunteer Ireland*, Dublin, (2017), https://www. volunteer.ie/wp-content/uploads/2017/08/Volunteer_Ireland-Report_ FINAL.pdf, page 5.

149. Alden, L.E. and Trew, J.L., 'If it makes you happy: Engaging in kind acts increases positive affect in socially anxious individuals', *Emotion*, (2013), 13(1), pages 64–75.

150. Tartakovsky, M., '5 tips for teaching your kids self-compassion',

PsychCentral.com, (2018), https://psychcentral.com/blog/5-tips-for-teaching-your-kids-self-compassion/.

151. Forman, F., *Self-kindness for kids: Whizzo-voice to the rescue!* Outside the Box Learning Resources, Co. Kildare, Ireland, (2019).

152. 'Mindfulness and Education: The 100 Hours, Mindfulness in schools', The 100 Hours.org, https://www.100hours.org/mindfulness.

153. Breslin, N., Coyne, M. and Quirke, S., *The Little Book of Sound*, A Lust for Life, Dublin, (2017), page 13.

154. as suggested by Louise Shanagher, www.louiseshanagher.com.

155. Nixon, R., '5 ways to foster self-compassion in your child', LiveScience. com, (2011), https://www.livescience.com/14144-parenting-tips-compassion-esteem.html.

156. Evans, J., *You can't MAKE children resilient!*, The Jane Evans.com, (2016), https://www.thejaneevans.com/you-cant-make-children-resilient/

157. Neuroscientist Professor Ian Robertson spoke about resilience in the RTÉ One 'Stressed' documentary, see video embedded in Coyne, M., 'Are we stressing our children out?', RTÉ Brainstorm, (2018), https://www.rte.ie/brainstorm/2018/0522/965272-are-we-stressing-our-children-out/.

158. In my quest to find out more about compassion-based resilience, I interviewed Fiona Brennan, clinical hypnotherapist and author of *The Positive Habit*.

159. Ibid.

160. Shobbrook-Fisher, Z., *Love in love out*, Go Mindfully.org, (2018), http://gomindfully.org/2018/12/10/love-in-love-out/.

161. Fiona Brennan.

162. Young, K., 'Anxiety in kids: How to turn it around and protect them for life', Hey Sigmund.com, adapted from https://www.heysigmund.com/anxiety-in-kids/.

163. Especially written for this book by Louise Shanagher.

164. Alexandra Koster adapted Daniel Siegel's Mindfulness meditation the 'Wheel of Awareness' into a visual format for children to use. Koster, A., *Roots and Wings: Childhood Needs a Revolution*. Roots & Wings Publishing, Ireland, (2018).

165. Pathways Health and Research Centre and Ministry of Children and Family Development FRIENDS for Life Program, 'Learning to think green thoughts/Changing unhealthy thoughts', Tools and Resources Stress Management, https://www.keltymentalhealth.ca/sites/default/files/documents/toolkit_for_families_-_changing_unhealthy_thoughts.pdf.

166. Young, K., 'Phobias and fears in children – Powerful strategies to try', Hey Sigmund.com, https://www.heysigmund.com/phobias-and-fears-in-children/.

167. Anxiety Canada Youth, 'Exposure: How to do it', Anxietycanada.com, https://youth.anxietycanada.com/make-list.

168. Anxiety BC Youth, 'Build your own fear ladder', Anxietycanada.com, https://youth.anxietycanada.com/sites/default/files/pdfs/Fear%20ladder.pdf.

169. List compiled with the help of Maria Dillon and Sinéad Ray, Assistant Psychologists.

A Word of Thanks

To Pete. My rock and best friend. I literally could not have done this without you, all the hours you put in for me and your gorgeous dinners. No one I'd rather spend my life and evenings in with. Two little monkeys, 22 years on and conversation still going … Superlike you x

Jessica Alice, gift from God, you light up our lives with your vibrant energy, dancing and smiles. Aimée Ann, beloved precious girl, your feistiness is adorable, as are your gorgeous loud smooches! I'm so proud of both of you and the little ladies you are becoming. Thanks for helping me to face my mammy wobbles and loving me every day despite them. So blessed to have you x

To my agent, Faith O'Grady. Thanks for taking a chance on me. Your unending support throughout really kept me going. Thanks for hooking me up with the perfect fit. To Eoin McHugh, publishing director at HarperCollins in Ireland. From the moment we met you just 'got' me and my idea, and it all flowed naturally from there. You're a true gentleman. To Nora Mahony, editor extraordinaire and unique KitKat eater! Thank you for turning my jumbled-up writing into something I'm really proud of. I'll miss our lovely Galway chats. To the HarperCollins in Ireland and UK teams, thanks for all of your support and guidance, especially Tony Purdue, Patricia McVeigh, Ciara Swift, Jacq Murphy, Mia Colleran, Mary Byrne, Ben Hurd, Claire Ward and Georgina Atsiaris.

To my beautiful mumsy and true friend, Patricia Lagendijk. I'll never forget writing this overlooking our amazing view, knowing you were close with me, always there as my anchor. To my daddy, Paul Lagendijk. Your support and encouragement were invaluable throughout the process and when I needed them most. Your inspirational morning texts just made my day. To my dancing queen sis, Ellen Lagendijk and family. Thanks for everything, pet. To my literary marvel bro, Paddy Lagendijk, and my amazing godson Idzi and family. Miss you guys. To Suzy, RIP. Cracked miss diva bum wiggles, you helped me appreciate the moments.

To my cousin Virginia O'Grady, RIP cuz. Such painfully beautiful memories of raucous laughter and devilment. To my auntie Joanie, such a lady. And to my cuz Hugh, proud of ya.

To Frank and Mary Coyne. Thank you for your always cosy welcomes and gourmet meals. You are wonderful grandparents to our girlies and have made me feel so at home. To Ann Coyne, RIP. Thank you for gifting me a peaceful writing den. We miss you loads. To Gerard Coyne. Coffee bud. For your warm company and for giving me a space to write. To Barbara Antelo. You're a ray of light. We're blessed to have you in our lives. To Mary Coyne Jr and family. So happy to have you in Ireland, sis. Thanks for being you. To Kevin Coyne and family. Ye rock. I hope to get into that 'inner circle' one of these days! To Joe Coyne and family and Frank Coyne Jr and family, always great company.

To Bernie Kelleher. Thank you for all your support to me and my parents over the years.

To my godfather, Guido Van De Kreeke, RIP, and my godmother Beata Welsing. Thank you.

To Caroline Maréchal Brodoux. Thanks for your amazing art work and proofreads, and for being my soul sister from our Seoul Cure teenage angst days to our Majorcan retirement. To more bloody good times! Nice?!

To my ward buddy and love warrior, Ruth Fagan. I always leave our chats feeling warm, grateful and inspired. So unbelievably happy our paths crossed. Love in … Love out! To my girl, Caitriona McMahon. It's only been five years and feels like a lifetime with you by my side. Thanks for your beautiful poem. Kayla, you rock too.

To Pamela Carroll Mannion. So happy to have you in my life, Sligo pal, sure where would I be without you? Thanks for our many lovely chats and your amazing contribution on CBT.

To Sinead Foran. I will always remember our Camden Street days. Lovely to still have you close by.

To Renette McLellan. Friend, teacher, tough-as-nails chick with a soft centre. Still like yesterday after 30 years. True friendship never dies. And your mummy is pretty cool too. To Nairi Hakhverdi, dearest childhood friend. Wishing you peace and love and remembering your beautiful mum Lilik too.

To June Harte. Beautiful soul inside and out. And to lovely Alma. Miss our Lady G. chats. To Sharon Jordan, Niamh Gill and Sonya Walsh. Forever the Fab Four. To Hazel Moore and girls. Gorgeous friend, 26 years on. Amazing our paths crossed again.

To Niamh Kennan, Matthew Bates and kids. Such brilliant forever friends. To Sofia Pettersson and Brian Gallen and girls. Our holiday buddies. So great knowing ye. To Grainne and Neil Griffin, Dee and Donie McFadden and girlies. Thanks for all your support. To all the school and neighbourhood parents, ye rock.

To Niall Breslin (Bressie). Good friend and kind hearted gentleman. Thanks for getting the ball rolling. And to all of you at A Lust for Life, #beproud, you're helping so many. To Susan Quirke. I remember talking to you about my 'dream'. Here it is! Thank you for being a shining light for humanity. So happy you're following your own star.

To Michelle Whelan Kennedy, of Galway Community Counselling. I've never felt so at home and at ease with a therapist. You welcome every part of me and for that I am truly grateful.

To Dr Roisin Joyce, of the Evidence-Based Therapy Centre, clinical supervisor and friend. Thank you for bringing me into the world of compassion – it has changed everything. To Aisling Leonard-Curtin. It's so lovely to support each other on our journeys. To Chris Winson. Thank you for your support and for bringing us #365daysofcompassion. To Dr Paul D'Alton, great to connect again after our Niteline years and thanks for your amazing endorsement of my book. To Dr Ciara Kelly, ballsy beauty, I really admire you. So grateful for your gorgeous Foreword.

To Nicole McGuigan, of Galway Parent Network. You have such a talent for reaching those in our community and beyond. Pleasure helping you to build happy babies everywhere. To my Early Years Committee, especially Evelyn Fanning, Morgan Mee, Linsey McNelis, Tara Durkin, Olwen Rowe, Aíne McNamara, Catherine Kinsella, Lisa Corbett, Ananda Geluk. So proud to be spreading awareness of infant mental health with you.

To Siobhán Prendiville, of the Children's Therapy Centre. Honoured your playful heart has a home in my book. And to my play therapy mummy, Eileen Prendiville, you're out of this world. To Louise Shanagher of Mindfully Me. I really admire your beautiful gentle spirit and your ability to reach into children's hearts. Thank you for your contribution.

To Fiona Brennan, of the Positive Habit. Thank you for sharing your wisdom. Your humanity, calm and positivity really shine through. To Sharon Fitzmaurice, angellically wild. To Hannah Lilly, kindred spirit bringing us #thejoyproject. To Alex Koster, mindfully seeing the beauty in children. To Caroline Foran, hugely talented writing buddy. To Sam Synnott, love what you do. To Brian Pennie, hell yeah!

To my fellow HarperCollins authors Brian O'Connell and Mike Hanrahan, Banner Legends and partners in divilment.

To Sabrina Crowe. We gotta clone you, as everyone needs a Sab in their lives! Thank you for everything you helped me with, you're a lifesaver. To Bébhinn Kelly, Ruth Shanahan, and all my amazing Doughiska colleagues, I could not ask for a sounder bunch. To my HSE Primary Care Psychology colleagues, really lovely to work with. To my NUIG Psychology colleagues, great memories, more to come. To Sinéad Ray. It was a dream to have you by my side. Thanks to you and Maria Dillon for your help on the Resources list. You'll both go very far!

To all those who have supported my journey along the way, thank you from the bottom of my heart.

To all my clients, old and new. Thank you for opening up your hearts to me and having hope in better days ahead. I hope you've gained a sense of how special and deserving you truly are.

To every child and grown-up child who feels anxious out there, this one's for *you*. I've been there, it's really hard – and I'm holding your hand. I hope this book gives you a voice and does you justice.